THE CELLULAR BASIS OF THE IMMUNE RESPONSE

THE CELLULAR BASIS OF THE IMMUNE RESPONSE

An Approach to Immunobiology

Edward S. Golub
PURDUE UNIVERSITY

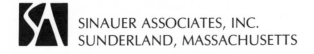 SINAUER ASSOCIATES, INC.
SUNDERLAND, MASSACHUSETTS

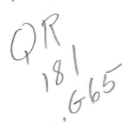

Second printing February 1978

Library of Congress Cataloging in Publication Data

Golub, Edward S   1934–
    The cellular basis of the immune response.

    Includes bibliographies and index.
    1. Immunology.   2. Immune response.   I. Title.
[DNLM: 1. Immunity, Cellular.   QW504 G629c]
QR181.G65   591.2'9   77-3728
ISBN 0-87893-210-0

This Book is For

JONATHAN & MARK & JONATHAN & MARK & JONATHAN & MARK & JONATHAN &

CONTENTS

PREFACE

This book has grown out of a course in immunobiology which I have taught at Purdue University for the past several years. The course attempts to present an up-to-date overview of the biology of the immune response. It is not a comprehensive course covering all aspects of immunology. The emphasis is on cell interactions and regulation, subjects which are in my own specialty, but it also covers a good amount of immunoglobulin structure and the generation of diversity. In teaching the course, I try to illustrate as many points as possible with experimental design, as well as to describe the rationale and, when possible, the historical sequence of the experiments. I've tried to do that as much as possible in this book as well as to catch the flavor of how science is done and convey it in as pleasant a manner as I can. In choosing the particular experiments to illustrate the points which I have decided to make, I will no doubt shock, anger, or insult many friends and colleagues. I apologize to them for my idiosyncratic views but hope that by the time they finish reading the text they will become converts.

I have attempted to keep names of individuals to a minimum in the text. Inclusion of many names works a hardship on students, so I have included only the names of a few individuals and apologize to my colleagues (and I hope still my friends) who were not mentioned. Please know that I thought of each of you as I left your name out.

It must be emphasized that this book is not intended to be a compendium of facts. It is intended as a sweeping overview of the experimental basis of modern cellular immunobiology. Practicing cellular immunologists will be familiar with everything which is covered. The book is intended for upper-division undergraduates, graduate students, medical students, and scientists working in other areas of biomedical research who wish to redeem their lost youth.

If the book is used as a text in a formal course, I highly recommend sending the students to the literature to read original papers since I could not give critical evaluation of data in this book.

Finally I thank the many friends and colleagues who read parts of the manuscript and made so many helpful suggestions or who were so helpful in discussions of interpretations of data and trends and in sharing unpublished data. Their names are listed below. Any shortcomings in the text are to be blamed on them. I take full credit for any value in this book.

Frank Adler, Bernard Amos, Dick Asofsky, Dick van Bekkum, Harvey Cantor, Max Cooper, Gus Cudkowicz, Tony Davies, Karel Dicke, Jeaninne Durdik, Dick Dutton, Ger van den Engh, Marc Feldmann, Dick Gershon, Joel Goodman, Mel Greaves, Howard Grey, George Jannosy, David Katz, Elaine McDaniel, Rick Miller, Av Mitchison, Andres Mulder, Peter Panfili, Ben Pernis, Jim Prahl, Martin Raff, Janet Roman, Larry Ruben, Jim Russell, Stu Schlossman, Eli Sercarz, Liz Simpson, Greg Siskind, George Snell, Osias Stutman, Jim Till, Dennie Toth, Mary Ann Wagner, Leon Wofsy, Ed Yunis, and Rolf Zinkernagel. My thanks also to the students of Biol. 537 at Purdue, Biol. 185 at UCLA, and Biochem. C55 at Northwestern who gave, often with brutal frankness, a student's view of the book. Special thanks to Patrick Nickoletti, Marge Ramirez, and Fran Selleck for suffering through the typing of the manuscript, to the staff at the Jackson Laboratory, Bar Harbor, Maine, for hospitality while I was writing, and to Andy Sinauer for holding my hand through the trauma of doing the book.

Edward S. Golub
Lafayette, Indiana
November, 1976

1

INTRODUCTION AND THE NATURE OF SELECTION IN THE IMMUNE RESPONSE

OVERVIEW

The study of immunology has its historical roots in clinical medicine. The word itself derives from the Latin *immunitas* which means freedom from a public service and later came to be used to indicate freedom from disease. The ancients realized that after exposure to disease or recovery from a disease an individual was less susceptible to that disease. The Chinese practiced a form of vaccination long before Jenner, and Jenner himself was able to vaccinate against smallpox not because of exact technical knowledge, but rather from the observation that milkmaids, who had scars of the pox on their hands from cow pox (an occupational hazard), had fewer scars on their faces from smallpox than the rest of the population.[1] The history of immunology is really the story of the elucidation of the mechanisms behind this freedom from disease through prior contact.

Ironically, this book will not deal very much with either disease or the freedom from disease. Immunologists have found in the last few decades that the study of model systems which are not harmful yield a more fruitful means of studying the mechanisms of immunity. We should emphasize right at the outset that the mechanisms which the body uses to react to harmful substances are the same that it uses in reacting against nonharmful substances. Indeed, this unity of

---

[1]The Dutch scientist-musician G. J. van den Engh has pointed out to me the likelihood that milkmaids were generally known to be something special. The number of milkmaids who are chased through fields singing "fa la la" in English folk tunes far exceeds that of scullery maids, nannies, or seamstresses.

1

mechanisms has made immunology a useful and attractive subject, since fundamental mechanisms about disease processes can be studied in the absence of disease. So in this book we will be talking about the response of animals, usually the mouse, to such distinctly nonpathogenic substances as sheep red blood cells, bovine serum albumin, and keyhole limpet hemocyanin. The characteristic that all these diverse substances have in common is that they are foreign to the animal they are injected into, and this is the key to the immune response. *The body recognizes substances that are foreign and makes specific responses against them.*

THE NATURE OF SPECIFICITY

We will see in the course of this text that the immune response can be loosely divided into two types, antibody formation and cell-mediated responses. All the phenomena we will be examining are the result of events occurring in and on cells. The predominant cell type in the immune response is the lymphocyte. The aspects of the immune response involved in antibody formation are generally referred to as HUMORAL and those involved in tissue reactions as CELLULAR. It will appear in some parts of this text that they are really separate and distinct kinds of phenomena, but this is not the case. To study something in science, one must isolate it from as many other factors as possible, and in doing this, the illusion of separateness is often maintained after the experiment is over. Because of this, one must always try to fit the isolated observation, or more accurately, the observation of the isolated, into a total picture. In the case of the immune response, the humoral and cellular aspects are really parts of a continuum of responses, and the cells and events involved in one may overlap the other. To study either, however, attention is focused on the particular one being studied.

The humoral aspect of the response refers to the producing of serum antibodies. When a foreign material—called an ANTIGEN—is injected into an animal, a complex series of events occurs. One result of these events is the appearance in the serum of molecules which can specifically combine with the antigen. These molecules are called ANTIBODIES. The antibody molecule is one of the best studied of protein molecules, and its structure and nature will be covered in detail in Section III. At this time it is important to emphasize only that in response to a specific antigen the animal responds with the production of proteins which can combine specifically with the antigen. Thus, if a mouse is injected with sheep red blood cells, after an interval there will appear in the serum antibodies which combine with the sheep red blood cells. These anti–sheep red blood cell antibodies will not react with horse red blood cells or bovine serum albumin. Now the very interesting point is that the molecules which have this specificity are of a type (gamma globulins) which are present in the serum at all times. It is not the production of a new *kind* of molecule that has been induced but rather of new combining *specificities* within the globulins. The specificity of these molecules will be shown to be due to differences in the sequence of amino acids in only a very small portion of the peptide chains making up the antibody molecule. Each specificity is coded for in the DNA of the cell producing the antibody since it is part of the dogma of modern biology that the order of amino acids in a peptide reflects the order of the nucleotides in the DNA of the cell which produced the peptide.

The antibodies mentioned above are produced by cells called LYMPHO-CYTES. Thus the study of the humoral part of the immune response is also the study of the cellular basis for antibody production since antibodies are produced by cells. But the lymphocytes can be sub-divided into at least two classes or types called B-CELLS and T-CELLS. One of these classes of lymphocytes, the B-cell, is responsible for the synthesis and secretion of antibody molecules. The other, the T-cell, is responsible for helping the B-cell do this, but T-cells are also able to carry out a whole series of reactions on their own. Generally these are reactions which involve tissue destruction. Since antibody is not involved in these reactions, they are called CELL-MEDIATED REACTIONS. Such reactions have the same (or very similar) ranges of specificity as do humoral reactions. That is to say, the tissue of an animal has chemical groupings which are antigenic in some other species and can therefore be recognized as foreign and reacted against. Instead of a reaction leading to antibody formation, however, the responding cells may react directly with the antigen on the foreign tissues and cause destruction of that tissue. Some current thinking about the body's defense against tumors is that a tumor has unique antigens and is therefore recognized as foreign. The immune system then responds against the new antigens, and in this manner there is constant immune surveillance against tumors. Failure to react with the new antigen results in cancer.

SELECTIVE VS. INSTRUCTIVE THEORIES OF THE IMMUNE RESPONSE

If, as we have said, there are cells which are able to produce antibodies of great specificity and there are cells able to react with tissues with an equal degree of specificity, it is very important to know how these cells interact with the specific antigen to initiate and carry out the processes. One school of current immunological thought has it that the elements of immunological specificity probably arose only in one form in the animal. That is to say, it is simplest to think that the manner in which an antibody molecule expresses its specificity must be the manner in which a lymphocyte expresses its specificity. Now if we accept this notion for the time being and argue that cell and product (antibody molecule) derive their specificity from a common mechanism, the next step in our reasoning is that the cell must have something like an antibody on its surface to react with antigen. The logic is pushed even further (on some experimental evidence which we shall look at in a later chapter) to say that the cells which will make antibodies of a given specificity have molecules of that antibody on their surfaces which act as *receptors* for antigen. Interaction between receptor and antigen somehow transmits a signal to the cell to produce more of the same antibodies and to divide. We know that the specificity of the antibody molecule is derived from one small portion of the peptide chain of the molecule; the argument thus runs that the genome of the cell producing the antibody has the genetic code for that particular sequence of amino acids which gives the molecule its specificity and that all the antibody molecules synthesized by that particular cell have that same sequence of amino acids and therefore that specificity. Once some fundamental assumptions are made, it really is an attractive hypothesis.

One prediction from the above theory is that there should be antibody molecules on the surface of lymphocytes to act as receptor sites for antigen. This turns out to be the case for B-cells (Chapter 5). One of the identifying characteristics of the B-cell is the presence of antibody, or more correctly immunoglobulin, molecules on the surface of these cells. But life is not all beer and skittles and the T-cell does not have nearly the quantity of immunoglobulin on its surface that the B-cell does. This fact is rather troublesome, and it has generated a good deal of controversy in recent years. The nature of the T-cell receptor is a fundamental problem in immunology and as of this time is still in doubt. One must therefore ask, if the T-cell has a receptor which expresses its specificity in a manner other than the manner of the immunoglobulin and the B-cell, do we now have to explain two separate mechanisms of specificity?

Whatever the nature of the receptor, the evidence seems quite convincing that there are lymphocytes reactive to a particular antigen present in the animal before it is challenged with antigen. When the animal is confronted with an antigen, the number of these specific cells rises rapidly, almost astronomically. The question is how? Paul Ehrlich (1854 to 1915) developed the first useful theory to answer this problem. Ehrlich was one of the first to suspect that the mysterious substances (antibodies) in the serum after disease or immunization were produced by cells, and he formulated a theory which is frighteningly up to date considering that it was put forth over fifty years ago. (Perhaps this tells us something about up-to-datedness. More likely it tells us that genius sees problems in unusual ways, whether the time for that view has come or not.) Ehrlich postulated that a cell had *side chains* and that these side chains were the serum substances, i.e., the antibodies. Each cell had a set of side chains which was a reflection of the responses which the animal could make. Thus, animals make antibodies against tetanus toxoid, and so there was a side chain for tetanus toxoid. Similarly, animals make a response against the organism which causes pneumonia, so there was a side chain for that organism. In modern jargon we would say that a given lymphocyte (cell) had an antibody molecule as a receptor (side chain) for each of the antibodies the animal could make. Ehrlich envisioned the antigen reacting with the specific side chain, and as a result of this interaction the other side chains disappeared and the cell began producing only the side chain with the specificity of the antigen. These side chains left the surface of the cell and appeared in the serum, thus raising the level (or titer) of serum antibody against the antigen. This concept is diagrammed in Figure 1.

This very clever theory stood for awhile, but the great immunochemist, Karl Landsteiner (1868 to 1943), produced evidence which led to the abandoning of the side chain theory. Landsteiner synthesized organic compounds and tested their ability to induce antibody or to react with antibodies made against similar molecules. He would synthesize a small molecule which, when attached to a large one, gave rise to antibodies directed against the small molecule. The small molecule was called a HAPTEN; the larger one to which it was attached, a CARRIER (or "schlepper"). When Landsteiner introduced an NO_2 group onto a benzene ring to make nitrobenzene as the hapten, he found that he could get specific antibody directed against the nitrobenzene. When he introduced two NO_2 groups to produce the dinitrobenzene hapten, he found that he got a specific antibody directed against that molecule. Similarly, if he added sulfonic acid or arsonic acid to the ring, he generated specific antibodies against these compounds. Well, how can one visualize a cell with specific side chains, each chain specific for a given antigen to which the animal can respond, if one can go into the laboratory and synthesize a

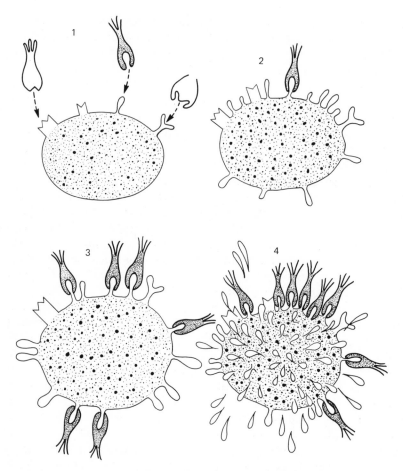

1

Paul Ehrlich's side-chain theory for antibody production. [From the original publication (1900). *Proc. Roy. Soc. B.* 66, 424.]

seemingly endless array of compounds? This discovery signaled the apparent end of the side-chain theory and introduced a new set of notions.

The side-chain theory really is a form of *selective theory*. Since the cell has the side chain, what is required is that it react with antigen and then more of the chains be produced. Thus the antigen selects the specific side chain. What followed was a novel move away from selective mechanisms to *instructive* theories of antibody formation. The leading proponents of these were Felix Haurowitz and then Linus Pauling in the 1940s and 1950s. Very briefly, the instructive theories of antibody formation postulated that a cell which makes an antibody molecule is indifferent to the specificity of the molecule. The machinery for the synthesis of proteins was then not at all understood, and the cell was visualized as being able to spin out a protein molecule and then to introduce some imprint into the molecule in the final stages. This final fillip to a jaded molecule gave it the specificity for interaction. We know now that the final shape of a protein molecule is determined by the primary sequence of the amino acids and that this sequence is a reflection of the DNA which codes for that protein. The DNA is transcribed into RNA, which is then used as a template in translation to string together the proper amino acids. Since secondary and tertiary structure depends on primary structure, the specificity must be built into the genetic code. But in the 1940s these facts were not known, and the proponents of the instructive theories of antibody formation visualized that a small fragment of antigen got into the cell and altered the shape of the peptide chain as it was being synthesized. Thus, antigen instructed the cell as to the nature of the specificity of the molecule it was to produce.[2] This theory is diagrammed in Figure 2.

[2]The instructive theory of antibody formation had a great influence on early molecular biology. The theory was so attractive that attempts to understand regulatory phenomena in microbial systems were cast in instructive terms. Only when molecular biologists arrived at the "trinity" (DNA, RNA, peptide) was this idea no longer used in both molecular biology and immunology. I thank the historian of science Dr. Robert Obley for this instructive insight.

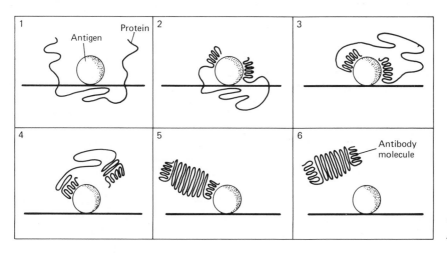

Linus Paulings's direct template theory. [From Pauling (1940). *J. Amer. Chem. Soc.* 62, 2643.]

As our knowledge of the mechanisms of protein synthesis in-creased and as it became increasingly difficult for the instruc-tionalists to explain certain aspects of the immune response (the secondary response and tolerance, in particular), there was a growing uneasiness with the theory and a casting about for an alternative. Niels Jerne, probably as a result of the influence of the phage group on his thinking, evolved a new incarnation of the selective theories called the NATURAL SELECTION THEORY. Here is Jerne's reminiscence about his insight.[3]

'Can the truth *(the capability to synthesize an antibody)* be learned? If so, it must be assumed not to pre-exist; to be learned, it must be acquired. We are thus confronted with the difficulty to which Socrates calls attention in Meno (Socrates, 375 B.C.), namely that it makes as little sense to search for what one does not know as to search for what one knows; what one knows one cannot search for, since one knows it already, and what one does not know one cannot search for, since one does not even know what to search for. Socrates resolves this difficulty by postulating that learning is nothing but recollection. The truth *(the capability to synthesize an antibody)* cannot be brought in, but was already inherent.'

The above paragraph is a translation of the first lines of Soren Kier-kegaard's "Philosophical Bits or a Bit of Philosophy" (Kierkegaard, 1844), By replacing the word "truth" by the italicized words, the statement can be made to present the logical basis of the selective theories of antibody formation. Or, in the parlance of Molecular Biology: synthetic potentialities cannot be imposed upon nucleic acid, but must pre-exist.

I do not know whether reverberations of Kierkegaard contributed to the idea of a selective mechanism of antibody formation that occurred to me one evening in March 1954, as I was walking home in Copenhagen from the Danish State Serum Institute to Amaliegade. The train of thought went like this: the only property that all antigens share is that they can attach to the combining site of an appropriate antibody molecule; this attachment must, therefore, be a crucial step in the sequences of events by which the introduc-tion of an antigen into an animal leads to antibody formation; a million structurally different antibody-combining sites would suffice to explain serological specificity; if all 10^{17} gammaglobulin molecules per ml of blood are antibodies, they must include a vast number of different combining sites, because otherwise normal serum would show a high titer against all usual antigens; three mechanisms must be assumed: (1) a random mechanism for ensuring the limited synthesis of antibody molecules possessing all possible combining sites, in the absence of antigen, (2) a purging mechanism for repressing the synthesis of such antibody molecules that happen to fit to auto-antigens, and (3) a selective mechanism for promoting the synthesis of

---

[3] As an interesting aside, when Jerne wrote this reminiscence he was director of the Paul Ehrlich Institute in Germany. This seems rather appropriate.

those antibody molecules that make the best fit to any antigen entering the animal. The framework of the theory was complete before I had crossed Knippelsbridge. I decided to let it mature and to preserve it for a first discussion with Max Delbrück on our freighter trip to the U.S.A., planned for that summer. [Niels K. Jerne, *The Natural Selection Theory of Antibody Formation; Ten Years Later,* In *Phage and the Origins of Molecular Biology,* Cold Spring Harbor Laboratory of Quantitative Biology, 1966, p. 301.]

In his NATURAL SELECTION THEORY Jerne visualized that a cell was programmed to make only one specificity of antibody and that it did this even in the absence of antigenic stimulus. Thus there would always be a low level of antibody in the serum. When antigen was introduced into the system, this antibody would react with the antigen, and the antigen-antibody complex would find its way back to the cell which originally produced the antibody. The interaction of the antigen-antibody complex with the cell now stimulated the cell to divide, and there were thus many more of these cells after a short time, all producing antibodies of that one specificity.

F. M. Burnet (later Sir MacFarlane Burnet) modified this theory into the CLONAL SELECTION THEORY, the theory that most immunologists function under today and which will be assumed to be true in most of the thinking in this book. According to the clonal selection theory, a cell is programmed in its DNA to make one or at best a very few specificities. Antigen reacts with receptors at the surface of these cells, and this reaction constitutes a signal for the cell to divide. After several rounds of multiplication these cells which have been selected by antigen are the dominant specificity of the lymphocytes in the body, and the antibody they produce is found in high concentration in the serum.

This is essentially the state that the study of immunology has reached today. Virtually all practicing immunologists adhere to a clonal selection theory of one shade or another. All agree that the response has specificity and that there is roughly a cellular and a humoral aspect with varying degrees of overlap. How then does the whole thing work? How does the animal prevent reactions against itself? What controls the response so that it ceases at some point? All this and more make up the field of immunobiology, and this book will attempt to go into the major experiments which have provided the current thinking.[4]

[4]One of the leading philosophers of science, Thomas Kuhn, in his book *The Structure of Scientific Revolutions* argues that science moves forward by changing *paradigms.* A paradigm is a commonly held belief among scientists. It need not be correct, merely accepted. Kuhn argues that all experiments are really designed to prove the paradigms. When enough data is generated so that the paradigm begins to be

READINGS

Burnet, F. M. (1959). *The Clonal Selection Theory of Immunity*. Nashville, Tenn., Vanderbilt University Press. (The basis of the current paradigms.)

Burnet, F. M. and Fenner, F. (1949). *The Production of Antibodies,* Melbourne, Macmillan. (The idea of self-nonself is beautifully developed here.)

Jerne, N. K. (1955). The natural selection theory of antibody formation, *Proc. Nat. Acad. Sci.* **41,** 849. (A critical idea paper that started the modern era.)

Jerne, N. K. (1967). Waiting for the end, *Cold Spring Harbor Symposium on Quant. Biol.* **32,** 591. (The state of the art in 1967 when it looked like the end was near.)

Landsteiner, K. (1936). *The Specificity of Serological Reactions,* Springfield, Ill., Thomas. (A classic.)

Lederberg, J. (1959). Genes and antibodies, *Science,* **129,** 1669. (A brilliant analysis by a nonimmunologist who is one of the founders of modern genetics.)

Pauling, L. (1940). A theory of the structure and process of formation of antibodies, *J. Am. Chem. Soc.* **62,** 2643. (An early, clear exposition of the direct template idea.)

GENERAL TEXTS

Eisen, H. (1974). *Immunology,* Hagerstown, Md., Harper & Row. (A masterful covering of all aspects of immunology.)

Fudenberg, H. H., Stites, D. P., Caldwell, J. L., and Wells, J. U. (1976). *Basic and Clinical Immunology,* Los Altos, Calif., Lange. (A good text with a clinical orientation.)

Good, R. A., and Fisher, D. W. (eds.) (1971). *Immunobiology,* Sunderland, Mass., Sinauer Associates. (A very good series of papers on many aspects of the immune response.)

Kabat, E. A. (1968). *Structural Concepts in Immunology and Immunochemistry,* New York, Holt, Rinehart and Winston. (A thorough covering of the structural basis of immunoglobulin and antigen binding.)

Kuhn, T. (1970). *The Structure of Scientific Revolutions,* 2nd ed., University of Chicago Press. (An extremely important book which presents the argument of changing paradigms.)

FOOTNOTE 4 (*Continued*)

less universally accepted, a new paradigm takes its place. This view of science is contrary to that of Karl Popper, who argues that scientists actually set out to disprove ideas. But whether Kuhn or Popper is more correct is not our prime concern. I have used Kuhn's notion of paradigms in selecting experiments to illustrate the developing thoughts of modern immunobiology. Regardless of *how* paradigms change, the fact remains that they *do* change, and I have tried to show the evidence which caused immunologists to adopt new paradigms.

Mazumdar, D. M. H. (1975). The purpose of immunity: Landsteiner's interpretation of the human isoantibodies, *J. Hist. Biol.* **8,** 115. (A very readable article by an historian showing the changing ideas of the study of the immune response.)

Roitt, I. M. (1971). *Essential Immunology,* Oxford, Blackwell Scientific Publications. (A readable overview of immunology with an orientation toward antibody and antibody-mediated hypersensitivity.)

I

LYMPHOCYTE POPULATIONS: B-CELLS AND T-CELLS

In this section we will show that both the antibody (humoral) and cell-mediated limbs of the immune response are brought about by interacting cell populations. Both forms of the immune response are carried out by cells with antigen specificity and cells without specificity. The cells with antigen specificity (those cells which are preprogrammed to react with certain antigens and not with others) are lymphocytes. The cells without specificity are macrophages. The lymphocytes and macrophages are derived from a primordial blood-forming cell called a pluripotent hemopoietic stem cell. All other cells of the blood, erythrocytes, granulocytes, and platelets, are also derived from the stem cell. Some unknown factors cause the stem cell to become committed to differentiate into a cell called a progenitor cell. The progenitor cell at some stage of its development becomes committed to differentiate into one of the types of blood cell. Differentiation of the committed progenitor cell occurs in the hemopoietic-inducing microenvironment (HIM).

The HIM for lymphocytes are the thymus and the equivalent of the bursa of Fabricius which in mammals is probably primarily the bone marrow. In these HIM the precursors differentiate into lymphocytes. There are two classes of lymphocytes: those which differentiate under the influence of the thymus, called thymus-derived lymphocytes (or T-cells), and those which differentiate in the bursal equivalent or bone marrow, called B-cells. Both B-cells and T-cells have characteristic antigens and receptors on their surface which serve as convenient means of identification.

13

Most important, however, is the fact that the lymphocyte populations carry out the specific phases of immune responses. In both humoral and cellular immune responses there is interaction between lymphocytes. In antibody formation there is B-cell:T-cell interaction. The B-cell is the precursor of the antibody-forming cell. However, for most antigens B-cells can't become effector cells (antibody-producing cells) unless they interact with T-cells. T-cells thus serve the capacity of being helper cells in antibody formation. In cell-mediated responses (graft rejection, graft-versus-host reactions, cell-mediated lympholysis) the effector cell is a T-cell. In cell-mediated responses, as in antibody formation, the precursor of the effector cell cannot become a functional effector cell without a helper cell. Thus, in cell-mediated responses one subpopulation of T-cells acts as the helper cell and one subpopulation of T-cells acts as the effector cell; in short, there is T-cell:T-cell interaction.

The key point of Section I is that lymphocytes interact with each other in a helper:effector relationship.

2

ORIGIN AND DISTRIBUTION OF LYMPHOID TISSUE

OVERVIEW

Immune reactions are carried out by lymphocytes. It is obvious that the various cells of the blood (erythrocytes, granulocytes, and lymphocytes) are very different from each other. They have different morphology and, more important, totally different functions. Because of these differences it might be natural to assume that they also have very different origins. This is not the case, however, and in this chapter we will examine some of the evidence showing that all the cells of the blood are derived from a common ancestral cell. It will become evident that the pattern of development for all cells of the blood is from pluripotent stem cell to progenitor cell to precursor of a functional end cell. The critical events of differentiation from progenitor cell to precursor cell occur in microenvironments. The lymphoid microenvironments are the thymus and the bursa. These are called primary lymphoid organs. Lymphocytes from these primary lymphoid organs are exported to the peripheral, or secondary, lymphoid organs. These are the spleen and lymph nodes.

ORIGIN OF THE CELLS OF THE BLOOD

Study of Hemopoiesis

The process of blood cell formation is called HEMOPOIESIS (*hemo* meaning blood, *poiesis* meaning formation). The fact that all the cells of the blood have finite life-spans but are constantly replenished argues that there must be a mechanism for their renewal. Whether each cell type has a separate renewal system or all derive from a common cell is one of the most interesting questions in biology and has obvious implications in medicine. One of the first major clues about the nature of the self-renewal system of blood cells came from studies in radiobiology in which it was found that the hemopoietic systems of an animal could be destroyed by X-irradiation. The entire system could be fully restored by injecting bone marrow or spleen cells from a compatible donor. It was clear from these studies that the bone marrow and spleen were hemopoietic organs, i.e. blood-forming organs. The problem then became how to study the cells in these organs which were responsible for regeneration of all the cells of the blood. One of the major obstacles in studying the cells involved in hemopoiesis was the lack of a good quantitive methodology. Such a method, called the SPLEEN COLONY FORMING ASSAY, was devised by Till and McCulloch in 1961 (Figure 1). The assay is performed by lethally X-irradiating mice and then injecting small numbers of syngeneic bone marrow or spleen cells (syngeneic cells are cells from mice of the same inbred strain). The X-irradiation destroys the animal's own blood-forming capacity, and the mouse becomes a "living test tube" in which the injected cells can grow. After about 7 days the spleens of these injected mice are found to contain visible, discrete nodules. There is a linear relationship between the number of cells injected and the number of nodules or colonies obtained. Each nodule represents a colony of cells which is derived from a single cell. The cell which gives rise to the colonies is called the colony forming unit or PLURIPOTENT HEMOPOIETIC STEM CELL. It is the stem cell which gives rise to the cells of the blood.

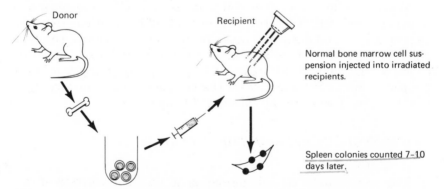

1

Normal bone marrow cell suspension injected into irradiated recipients.

Spleen colonies counted 7–10 days later.

Assay for spleen colony forming units (hemopoietic stem cells). [After Till and McCulloch (1961). *Rad. Res.* 14, 213.]

Nature of the Spleen Colonies

Histological examination of the colonies reveals that when they first are detectable (at about 4 days after injection) they are usually composed of one cell type, either erythroid *or* granuloid cells. This would be consistent with the idea that each of these blood cells has its own renewing cell system. However, by day 6 as many as 10 percent of the colonies contain mixtures of erythroid *and* granuloid cells. The number of mixed colonies increases with time until by day 12 as many as 47 percent of the colonies have more than one cell type. Mixed colonies are consistent with the idea that the different blood cells arise from the same cell; in other words, a single stem cell gives rise to erythroid and granuloid cells. An example of the composition of colonies is given in Table 1.

Proof of Single-Cell Derivation

Mixed colonies could be due to a common ancestral stem cell or two ancestral cells lodging in the same place in the spleen and giving rise to two colonies in one area. The fact that the slope of the titration curve (Figure 2) is linear provides a good argument that a single cell gives rise to a single colony. However, one would like to have an experimental testing of this notion. To do this, one needs a way of identifying the cells in the colony to see if they were the progeny of one stem cell or more than one stem cell. In turn, this requires that the cells must have a heritable, identifiable marker. If the stem cell had such a marker and all the cells in the colony also had it, the case would be strong for one stem cell giving rise to many cell types. On the other hand, if the cells in the colony were a mixture of cells with the marker and cells without the marker, then a strong case could be

TABLE 1. COMPOSITION OF SPLEEN COLONIES AFTER REPOPULATION WITH BONE MARROW CELLS.

Days after repopulation	Erythroid %	Granuloid %	Megakary %	Undifferen- tiated, %	Mixed %
4	66	22	0	12	0
6	59	23	1	7	10
7	60	22	3	0	15
8	51	20	14	5	10
9	52	17	10	5	16
12	31	10	12	0	47

Data from Currey and Trentin (1976). *Dev. Biol.* **15**, 395.

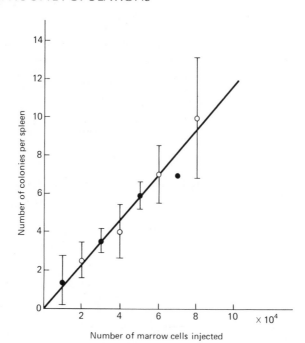

2

The relationship between the number of nucleated cells injected and the number of colonies formed in the spleen. [From Till and McCulloch (1961). *Rad. Res.* **14,** 213.]

made for more than one stem cell being responsible for the colony. A heritable, identifiable characteristic can be obtained by using *radiation-induced chromosome markers.* If mice are given sublethal X-irradiation (*ca.* 650 R), chromosomal abnormalities are induced in a small proportion of the cells. These chromosomal or karyotypic abnormalities are nonlethal and are passed on to the daughter cells. Bone marrow cells from mice with these markers are injected into lethally irradiated recipient mice which do not have the marker, and the cells in the colonies which develop are examined for the presence of the marker. If the colony develops from a single cell, then all the cells in the colony will have the unique chromosome marker. However, if the cells in the colony derive from different stem cells, then one-half to one-third of the cells should have the marker.

When this experiment was carried out, it was found that in those colonies which did have marked cells between 95 and 99 percent of the metaphase cells in day-11 colonies and between 83 and 98 percent of metaphase cells in day-14 colonies had the marker. This is highly suggestive evidence that the different cell types in the colony all come from a single stem cell.

A critical look at the data from the above experiment shows that as many as 17 percent of the cells in a colony did not have the marker. To answer the questions thus raised, a very complex series of experiments was designed and carried out to examine the percent of cells in metaphase with the marker and compare this value with the percent of metaphase cells which are erythroid and granuloid. The results of these experiments also strongly suggested that the colonies, and hence the erythrocytes, granulocytes, and megakaryocytes, derive from a single stem cell.[1]

Origin of Progenitor Cells in the Immune System

Just as repopulating lethally irradiated mice with compatible bone marrow cells restores their hemopoietic function, it also restores their immune function. The question then becomes, does the pluripotent stem cell also give rise to lymphocytes? In all the previous discussion we did not mention lymphocytes in the spleen colonies. Lymphocytes, in fact, do not appear in the colonies but rather are diffusely spread in the white pulp of the spleen by days 12 to 14 after repopulation with bone marrow cells. This could mean that lymphocytes do not derive from the pluripotent hemopoietic stem cell or that they do derive from the stem cell but cannot grow in the colonies.

Even though lymphoid cells cannot be found in the colonies, experiments using the chromosome marker techniques have shown that lymphoid cells are derived from the pluripotent hemopoietic stem cell. In experiments very similar to those described in the previous section, chromosome markers were induced in donors by means of nonlethal X-irradiation, and bone marrow from these mice was injected into lethally irradiated hosts. Later the lymphocytes of the thymus were examined to determine if they contained the unique marker. It was noted that the same marker found in lymphocytes was found in spleen colonies of the bone marrow used to repopulate these mice. Since the same unique marker appears in the lymphocyte and in the spleen colonies, this is a strong argument that the lymphocyte is derived from the stem cell.[2]

---

[1] The actual experiment involves passage of the cells into a mutant mouse called W/Wᵛ which cannot generate its own colonies. Details of the experiment are to be found in Wu *et al.* (1967). *J. Cell. Physiol.* **69,** 177.

[2] This is an oversimplification of the experiment. The actual experiment involved the W/Wᵛ mouse (see the preceding footnote).

Progenitor Cells and Hemopoietic-Inducing Microenvironments

The pluripotent hemopoietic stem cell, as we have seen, is assayed for by the *in vivo* colony forming cell assay. Another set of assays, carried out *in vitro,* determines the number of PROGENITOR CELLS. Progenitor cells are the first differentiated progeny of the stem cell. Unlike the stem cell, which is not responsive to inducing factors, the progenitor cell *is* responsive to these hormone-like substances which in some unknown manner induce cells to differentiate. There are also other differences between stem cells and progenitor cells. The stem cell is a resting cell while the progenitor cell actively synthesizes DNA. The progenitor cell is larger than the stem cell, and the two cells have at least one surface antigen which is different. The progenitor cell is much less well studied than the stem cell because only recently have good quantitative methods been developed for studying its function.

There are a variety of hormone-like substances which can act upon the progenitor cell and induce it to differentiate along a certain path toward becoming an identifiable functional cell. These substances are thought to be localized in anatomic microenvironments called HEMOPOIETIC-INDUCING MICROENVIRONMENTS (HIM). When the progenitor cell arrives at the appropriate HIM, it is acted upon by the hormone(s) of that microenvironment, and it begins to differentiate. For example, if the erythroid progenitor migrates to an erythroid-inducing microenvironment, it will be acted on by *erythropoietin* and begin to differentiate along a path leading to erythrocytes. Similarly, if the thymocyte progenitor cell migrates to the thymus, it will be acted on by *thymopoietin* and begin to differentiate to a thymic lymphocyte. Mixed colonies are thought to be colonies which develop at a juncture of two microenvironments. It appears that the progenitor cells for any cell type are committed to differentiate along a certain pathway. This pre-commitment to a form of differentiation is called DETERMINATION. Nothing is known about the way in which a cell becomes determined.

Progenitor cells for granulocytes are measured by an *in vitro* assay in which bone marrow or spleen cells are cultured on a thin layer of agar with a bizarre mixture of nutrients, which may include pregnant mouse uterus extract or factors from human urine, added to the cultures. These added materials are called COLONY-STIMULATING FACTOR(S) (CSF); little is known of their mode of action except that one or more are needed for *in vitro* growth and differentiation of granuloid progenitor cells. Under very stringent conditions, colonies develop on the agar which, when examined microscopically, are seen to be composed of granulocytes of varying degrees of maturity. For erythroid differentiation from progenitor cells, the hormone *erythropoietin* is added rather than colony-stimulating factor, and colonies of erythrocytes and their precursors develop. As a general rule the bone marrow contains 10 times as many granuloid and erythroid progenitors as does the spleen. To quantitate the number of thymocyte progenitor cells, bone marrow cells are treated with thymopoietin *in vitro,* and characteristic surface changes are measured.

Lymphocyte-Inducing Microenvironments

We have already developed the evidence that the lymphocytes are derived from the same stem cell as the erythrocytes and granulocytes. The microenvironments for erythroid and granuloid development are in the bone marrow and the spleen. There are at least two lymphocyte-inducing microenvironments. This is worth noting since we will very soon be developing the argument that there are two functional types of lymphocytes, thymus-derived and bursa- or bone marrow-derived. The microenvironment for the induction of thymus-derived lymphocytes is the *thymus*. The location of the second microenvironment is known in birds to be the *bursa of Fabricius,* but its location in mammals is not known. In mammals the bursa-equivalent seems to be diffusely spread throughout the hemopoietic organs (bone marrow and perhaps spleen). The thymus has two major cell types, lymphocytes and epithelial cells, and the factors which induce progenitor cells to differentiate into thymic lymphocytes are secreted by the epithelial cells. There are two possible candidates for the bursa-equivalent HIM. One is the GUT-ASSOCIATED LYMPHOID TISSUE (GALT), and the other consists of cells dispersed through the spleen and bone marrow. The evidence for either or both of those as sites of inducing activity is far from compelling.

In recent years there have been two candidates for the factor produced in the thymus which is reponsible for thymic lymphocyte differentiation. One of these is called THYMOSIN, which is an extract of thymus that has been subjected to several chemical enrichment procedures. The other is called THYMOPOIETIN, and it is also an extract of thymus, but it has been extensively purified and analyzed so that its amino acid sequence is known. Furthermore, thymopoietin has been solid-phase synthesized so that a synthetic product is available. A small number of cells in the bone marrow, when treated with either of these two products, undergo surface changes which we associate with thymic lymphocytes.

PRIMARY AND SECONDARY LYMPHOID TISSUE

It is generally thought that the progenitor cell migrates from the bone marrow via blood to either the thymus or the bursa-equivalent. When it arrives in the anatomical site, it is acted upon by the proper hormone-like factors (thymosin or thymopoietin in the thymus, an unknown substance in the bursa-equivalent). The progenitor then undergoes differentiative changes which cause it to become a morphologically recognizable lymphocyte. The organs in which the progenitor cells become converted into lymphocytes and which contain identifiable but predominantly nonfunctional lymphocytes are called the PRIMARY LYMPHOID ORGANS. In mammals these organs are the thymus and the bone marrow. Even though over 90 percent of the cells in the thymus have the morphological characteristics and many of the surface properties of lymphocytes, they cannot carry out the functions of known thymic-derived lymphocytes. This means that the vast majority of lymphocytes in the primary lymphoid organ are not functional cells.

Lymphocytes leave the primary lymphoid organs and take up residence in the SECONDARY LYMPHOID ORGANS where they are functional. In mammals the secondary lymphoid organs are the spleen and lymph nodes. The secondary organs contain mixtures of thymus- and bursa-derived lymphocytes in identifiable arrangements, but most important, the lymphocytes of secondary lymphoid tissue are able to carry out immune functions.[3]

SUMMARY

1. All the cells of the blood (erythrocytes, granulocytes, platelets, and lymphocytes) are derived from a common ancestral cell. This cell is called the pluripotent hemopoietic stem cell.

2. Pluripotent hemopoietic stem cells are assayed by their ability to form spleen colonies after being injected into lethally irradiated mice.

3. The colonies, which are derived from a single cell, contain mixtures of erythroid and granuloid cells. Chromosome marker experiments show that both of those cell types are derived from the same ancestral cell.

4. Chromosome marker experiments show that lymphocytes also are derived from the pluripotent hemopoietic stem cell, even though lymphocytes are not found in the colonies.

5. The stem cell is a metabolically inactive cell, but it differentiates into an actively metabolizing cell called the progenitor cell. The progenitor cell is

[3]Details of thymus-derived and bursa-derived lymphocyte function will be covered in Chapter 3.

responsive to hormone-like factors which induce the progenitor cell to begin to differentiate into functional cells.

6. The granuloid progenitor and erythroid progenitor cells are assayed by growth and differentiate in response to the proper factors added *in vitro.*

7. The progenitor cell is acted upon by the hormone-like inducing factors in certain anatomical sites. These are called hemopoietic-inducing microenvironments (HIM).

8. The HIM for lymphocytes are the thymus and the bone marrow which are called primary lymphoid organs. Lymphoid progenitor cells are acted upon by thymic HIM factors (thymosin or thymopoietin) and become thymocytes. The factors in the bone marrow are not known.

9. Lymphocytes leave the primary lymphoid organs and migrate to the secondary lymphoid organs. These are the spleen and lymph nodes.

10. Lymphocytes in the primary lymphoid organs are not able to carry out immune functions. Cells in the secondary lymphoid organs are functional cells.

READINGS

TEXT

Metcalf, D., and Moore, M. A. S. (1971). *Haemopoietic Cells,* Amsterdam, North-Holland Publishing Co. (A complete treatise on cfu-s and cfu-c.)

ARTICLES

Till, J. E., and McCulloch, E. A. (1961). A direct measurement of the radiation sensitivity of normal mouse bone marrow cells, *Radiat. Res.* **14,** 213.

Bradley, T. R., and Metcalf, D. (1966). The growth of mouse bone marrow cells *in vitro, Aust. J. Exp. Biol. Med. Sci.* **44,** 287.

(These two papers describe the methods of enumerating cfu-s and cfu-c.)

Wu, A. M., Till, J. E., Siminovitch, L., and McCulloch, E. A. (1967). A cytological study of the capacity for differentiation of normal hemopoietic colony forming cells, *J. Cell. Physiol.* **69,** 177.

————, ————, ————, and ———— (1968). Cytological evidence for a relationship between normal hematopoietic colony-forming cells and cells of the lymphoid system, *J. Exp. Med.* **127,** 455.

(These two papers contain experiments which show that the various end cells are derived from a common stem cell.)

3

CELL INTERACTIONS IN ANTIBODY FORMATION

OVERVIEW

Removal of the primary lymphoid organs (thymus and bursa) results in impaired immune responses. Neonatal thymectomy results in loss of ability to generate both antibody and cell-mediated responses, but neonatal bursectomy results in only a loss of antibody-forming potential. These findings have led to the notion of division of labor among lymphocytes. Repopulation of lethally irradiated mice with thymus cells or bone marrow cells alone does not restore their ability to make antibody, but injecting bone marrow and thymus cells together does reconstitute immune potential. Thus there is cellular cooperation in generating antibody responses. Repopulation of neonatally thymectomized mice with allogeneic thymus cells showed that the thymus cells were not producing antibody but that their presence was necessary to enable some cells already present in the host to generate antibodies. In experiments involving reconstitution of bone marrow and thymus of irradiated recipients, it was shown that the bone marrow cell becomes the antibody-producing cell. Thus the thymus-derived lymphocyte acts as a "helper" cell and the bone marrow-derived cell as the antibody-producing cell. A third, nonlymphoid, cell, the macrophage, is also required for immune functions. We see then that three cells, thymus-derived T-cells, bone marrow-derived B-cells, and macrophages, are needed for antibody formation.

24

DISCOVERY OF THYMUS- AND BURSAL-DERIVED LYMPHOCYTE FUNCTIONS

Effect of Neonatal Thymectomy

In the last chapter we showed that lymphocytes arise from the pluripotent hemopoietic stem cell through the action of inducing factors in the lymphocyte-inducing microenvironments. These lymphocyte-inducing microenvironments are the primary lymphoid organs, the thymus and the bursal equivalent (primarily the bone marrow). The modern era of the study of the cellular basis of the immune response can be looked upon as beginning with the simultaneous but independent observations on the role of the thymus by Robert A. Good in Minneapolis and J. F. A. P. Miller in England. Good, an immunologist and clinician, noted that in patients with thymomas (tumors of the thymus) there are often disorders of the immune system, especially acquired hypogammaglobulinemia (a severe reduction in the concentration of serum immunoglobulins). He and his colleagues carried out a very large series of experiments in which the thymus was removed from experimental animals, and the effect of this *thymectomy* on the immune response studied. Miller, working in London, was studying lymphocytic leukemia in mice. Because the thymus was known to be the target organ of the disease, he asked what the effect of removal of the thymus would be. He showed that in the absence of the thymus the mice did not develop leukemia, but he also saw that the removal of the thymus had very far-reaching implications on the immune response.

Both of these investigators found that removal of the thymus of mice within the first days after birth (neonatal thymectomy) resulted in a severe reduction in immune potential. When the neonatally thymectomized mice reached several weeks of age, they were either given skin from mice of other strains to test their ability to reject skin grafts or injected with antigen to test their ability to produce antibody. The neonatally thymectomized mice failed to reject skin grafts or produce antibody, while sham-thymectomized controls both rejected their grafts and produced antibody. Thymectomy of adult animals had only a marginal effect on either antibody responses or graft rejection. If the neonatally thymectomized mice were repopulated with thymocytes when they reached several weeks of age, their ability to generate antibody responses was restored.[1]

---

[1]The various methods and procedures used to measure immune responses are covered in Appendix I. The reader who is totally unfamiliar with antigen-antibody reactions would probably benefit from a reading of that section before proceeding.

Both men came to the same basic conclusion, that the thymus is of crucial importance in generating immune responses. Their pioneering work can be looked upon as the foundation of modern cellular immunobiology.

Effect of Bursectomy

The bursa of Fabricius is a lymphoid organ in the cloacal region of the chicken. Removal of this organ at birth also leads to impaired immune function. This remarkable and important discovery was made in 1954 by Bruce Glick, a graduate student at Ohio State University, who was attempting to find a possible function for the bursa. Here he relates how he discovered that the bursa plays a role in the immune response.

Up to the summer of 1954, bursectomy experiments had failed to reveal a specific function for the bursa. At this time nine of my 6-month-old experimental birds were used by Timothy S. Chang, a fellow graduate student, in a class demonstration which consisted of injecting chickens with *Salmonella typhimurium* O antigen and then determining the antibody titer of the serum. Six of the birds died immediately after the injection. Three survived, but to our surprise, their sera produced no agglutination when mixed with the homologous antigen. The wing-band numbers were checked with the record book, which revealed that all nine birds had previously been bursectomized. It appeared that the bursa was responsible for the results since the normal pen mates reacted to the injections by producing normal antibody titers. [Bruce Glick (1954). *The Thymus In Immunobiology,* p. 348.]

This rather startling result meant that either thymectomy or bursectomy could cause a severe depression of immune potential. It was soon found, however, that removal of the bursa did not impair the immune response in the same manner as did thymectomy. After neonatal thymectomy both graft rejection and antibody responses (cellular and antibody responses) were depressed. After neonatal bursectomy, however, antibody responses were depressed, but skin graft rejection was normal. This was found by showing that bursectomized chickens rejected grafts as well as sham-operated controls. These facts were a major piece of evidence which led to the insight that there is *division of labor among lymphocyte populations.*

EVIDENCE OF COOPERATING CELL POPULATIONS

In the early 1960s the picture which was emerging from the thymectomy and bursectomy studies showed that there was division of labor within the lymphocyte population. The bursa (or its equivalent in mammals) appeared to control some aspect of antibody formation, while the thymus appeared to be involved in both antibody formation and homograft reactions.

Bone Marrow-Thymus Reconstitution Experiments

The almost universal view of the thymectomy studies was that the thymus, the primary lymphoid organ, was seeding the secondary tissues with functional cells. This comforting notion was shaken by experiments from at least two sources which showed that the situation might not be this simple. This is another interesting case of two groups, one in America and one in England, doing experiments of different design but coming to the same important conclusion about a fundamental phenomenon.

In one set of experiments carried out by Claman and his co-workers in Denver, it was shown that repopulating lethally X-irradiated mice with thymus cells did not restore immune competence. The prediction, based on the accepted view of the day, was that if the thymus is seeding the secondary lymphoid organs with functional cells, then repopulating a mouse with thymocytes should restore its immune potential. The outline of this experiment is seen in Figure 1.[2] In this experiment the thymus and bone marrow of normal mice are removed and made into single-cell suspensions. An aliquot of each of the two populations is then injected into groups of lethally X-irradiated syngeneic recipients. Marrow and thymus are injected into one group, only thymus into another group, and only marrow into the third group. In this way the experiment has the necessary experimental and control groups to determine if either population alone produces antibody or if the two populations must both be injected. The mice are challenged with antigen [sheep red blood cells (SRBC)], and at an appropriate interval the amount of antibody produced is determined.

It can be seen from the experiment in Figure 1 that repopulating irradiated mice with either marrow alone or thymus alone was not sufficient to generate a significant titer of antibody. However, injecting cells from *both* of the primary lymphoid organs resulted in restoration of the antibody response. This showed clearly that thymus cells alone were not able to reconstitute the antibody response and immediately opened to question the view that the thymus exports all the functional cells in immune responses.

The second kind of experiment which raised doubt that all im-

---

[2]This study is a typical cell transfer experiment used in cellular immunology. It will be of great advantage to the reader to make sure that it is completely understood because this format will appear throughout the book.

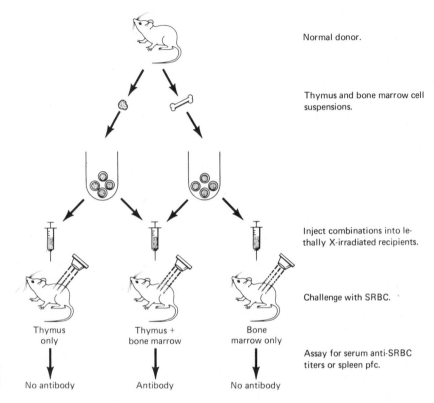

Normal donor.

Thymus and bone marrow cell suspensions.

Inject combinations into lethally X-irradiated recipients.

Challenge with SRBC.

Thymus only

Thymus + bone marrow

Bone marrow only

Assay for serum anti-SRBC titers or spleen pfc.

No antibody

Antibody

No antibody

1

Bone marrow–thymus reconstitution experiment. [After Claman, Chaperon, and Triplett (1969). _J. Immunol._ 97, 828.]

mune function was due to the cells of the thymus was done by Davies and his co-workers in London. They used cells with unique chromosome markers. In these experiments, mice were lethally irradiated and repopulated with either bone marrow or thymus cells. The mice used in these experiments had a naturally occurring chromosome marker similar to those which were induced in the studies in Chapter 2. By use of this marker it was possible to show that thymus cells proliferated in response to antigen but did not make antibody. Bone marrow cells injected into recipients which then received antigen but no thymus cells neither proliferated nor produced antibody. But when bone marrow and thymus cells were injected together and challenged with antigen, antibody was produced. So this experiment, like the one above, shows that thymus cells alone do not restore irradiated animals but combination of thymus and bone marrow do.

These two experiments showed that there were at least two lymphocyte populations involved in antibody formation and that some form of *cellular cooperation* was occurring between them. From these experiments it is also seen that the cells of the primary lymphoid organs (thymus and bone marrow) do not produce antibody by themselves, but when they are both injected into irradiated hosts, antibody is produced. The inescapable conclusion from these experiments is that there is cellular cooperation between bone marrow and thymus cell population and one or both of them were then able to produce antibody. The question then became which cell population was producing the antibody, the cells derived from the thymus or the cells derived from the bone marrow, or both.

IDENTIFYING THE EFFECTOR AND THE HELPER CELLS

Reconstitution after Neonatal Thymectomy

Because repopulation of neonatally thymectomized mice with thymus cells reconstituted the ability of these mice to produce antibody against SRBC, it was assumed that the thymus lymphocytes were the eventual antibody-forming cells. The bone marrow-thymus reconstitution experiments, however, suggested that cooperation was occurring between the thymus and bone marrow cells, and from the experiments with chromosomally marked cells it was suggested that the thymus-derived cells were not the ones producing antibody. It then became crucial to definitively determine which cell was producing the antibody and what the other cell type was doing.

The experiment which gave the first clear answer to this question was performed by G. F. Mitchell and Miller and is one of exceptional elegance. Needed in this experiment are readily identifiable markers for the cells of the thymus-derived population and another set of markers for the cells of the bone marrow-derived population. Such markers exist in the form of genetically controlled surface antigens of the major histocompatability complex on cells. These antigens are called HISTOCOMPATABILITY ANTIGENS or H-2 antigens (for a detailed discussion of H-2 see Chapter 6). Mice of the same inbred strain all have the same H-2 antigens on their cell surfaces, but mice of another strain may have a different set of H-2 antigens. For example, mice of the CBA strain have one set of antigens, and C57BL/6 mice have another set. Because the CBA strain has H-2 antigens which C57BL/6 does not have, if CBA cells are injected into C57BL/6, they will be recognized as foreign and C57BL/6 will produce antibodies directed against the H-2 antigens on the CBA cells. Thus one can produce antibodies which will react with CBA cells that in the presence of complement will lyse these cells (see Appendix I). By injecting CBA mice with C57BL/6 cells, an anti-C57BL/6 serum can be produced. In fact, by immunizing proper strains, one can produce reagent antisera against all the H-2 types. This procedure is graphically demonstrated in Figure 2. When C57BL/6 anti-CBA antiserum (i.e., an antiserum produced by C57BL/6 against cells of CBA) is reacted with cells from a CBA mouse, there is a reaction of the anti-H-2 antibodies with the H-2 antigen molecules on the cell surface. The addition of complement causes the cells to lyse. Therefore one has a marker for cells of a given H-2 specificity and can eliminate the cells with the marker from a population. This is seen graphically in Figure 3.

The idea of the Mitchell-Miller experiment was to repopulate a

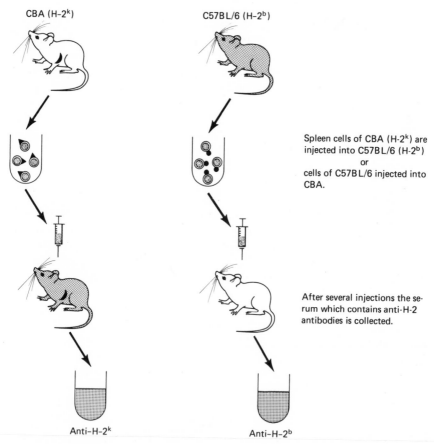

CBA (H-2^k)

C57BL/6 (H-2^b)

Spleen cells of CBA (H-2^k) are injected into C57BL/6 (H-2^b)
or
cells of C57BL/6 injected into CBA.

After several injections the serum which contains anti-H-2 antibodies is collected.

2

Anti-H-2^k

Anti-H-2^b

Production of anti-H-2 antibody.

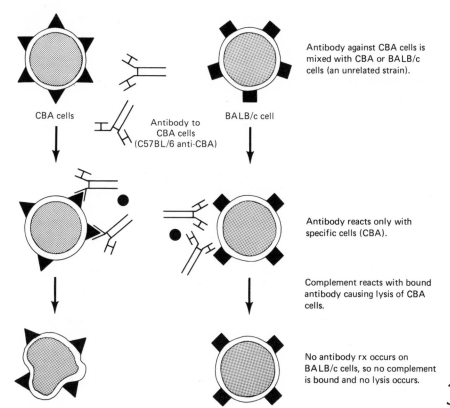

CBA cells

Antibody to
CBA cells
(C57BL/6 anti-CBA)

BALB/c cell

Antibody against CBA cells is
mixed with CBA or BALB/c
cells (an unrelated strain).

Antibody reacts only with
specific cells (CBA).

Complement reacts with bound
antibody causing lysis of CBA
cells.

No antibody rx occurs on
BALB/c cells, so no complement
is bound and no lysis occurs.

3

Inhibition of antibody-forming cells by anti-H-2 antibodies.

neonatally thymectomized mouse of one H-2 type, after it had reached
8 weeks of age, with thymus cells from a mouse of another H-2 type.[3]
This will restore the ability of the thymectomized animal to produce
antibody-forming cells against SRBC. The crucial part is to then
determine which H-2 antigens are on the surface of the antibody-
producing cells. If they are the same as those of the injected thymus
cells, then this shows that the thymus-derived cells are the cells
which produce antibody. If they are not the same H-2 as the injected
thymus cells but of the type of the thymectomized host, then this
shows that a cell already present in the host is producing the
antibody but was unable to do so until the thymus cells were present.

[3]Cell transfer experiments using mice of the same H-2 antigen are called
ISOGENEIC. If cells of different H-2 types are used, the transfer is called ALLOGENEIC. If
cells of different species are used, e.g., rat or human cells injected into mice, the
transfer is called XENOGENEIC.

The anti-H-2 antiserum is used to determine the H-2 type of the antibody-forming cells. Since anti-H-2 antibody which has reacted with cells with the appropriate H-2 antigen on their surfaces will allow complement to bind to the AgAb complex, these cells will be lysed in the presence of complement and will no longer be able to carry out any function. If these cells are antibody-producing cells, then the number of antibody-producing cells in the population will be drastically reduced. The appropriate controls for this experiment are to react the cells with an antiserum which contains antibodies against some H-2 antigens other than those on the cell surface and also with normal serum which contains no anti-H-2 antibodies.

When this experiment was carried out, as in Figure 4, it was found that there was no reduction in antibody-producing cells after treatment of the cells of the repopulated animals with antibodies directed against the H-2 of the injected thymus cells. However, there was almost complete abolition of the antibody-forming cells after treatment with an antiserum directed against the cells of the neonatally thymectomized host. This experiment shows that the thymus cells are not becoming antibody-producing cells but that some cell type already present in the neonatally thymectomized mouse is now able to become an antibody-forming cell. It also shows that the presence of the thymus cell is required for the host cell to become an antibody-forming cell. In other words, the thymus cell acts as a "helper" cell for some other cell to become an effector cell or antibody-forming cell.

Bone Marrow-Thymus Reconstitution Experiments

Having shown that the thymus-derived cells act as helper cells but do not become antibody-producing cells, the next logical step was to determine if the effector cells, the antibody-producing cells, were cells from the other primary lymphoid organ, the bone marrow. The experiment seemed simple to do, merely to carry out the marrow-thymus reconstitution experiment (as diagrammed in Figure 1 in Chapter 3) with bone marrow of one H-2 type donor and thymus of another H-2 type and treat the antibody-forming cells with anti-H-2 antiserum as in Figure 3 of Chapter 2. Surprisingly, when the first part of this experiment was attempted (the allogeneic reconstitution), it was found that no antibody-forming cells could be generated when bone marrow and thymus cells were of different H-2 types. In other words, attempts at allogeneic marrow-thymus interactions were unsuccessful. This is an important fact, and we will return to it with great emphasis in Chapter 9, but the problem still remained to determine if the bone marrow cells were the cells producing antibody.

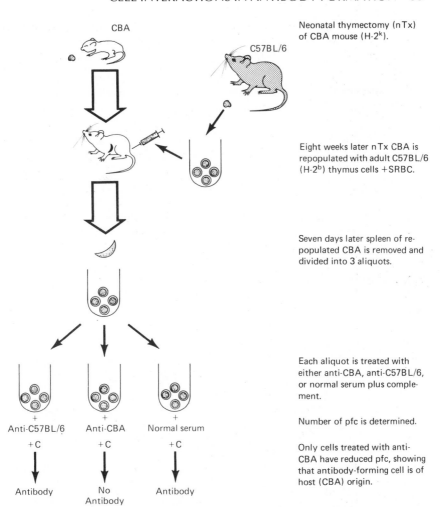

Determining if thymus cells become antibody-forming cells. [After Mitchell and Miller (1968). *P.N.A.S.* **59**, 296.]

To do the experiment, advantage was again taken of markers, but this time of chromosome markers, not cell surface markers. There is a mutant of the CBA mouse which has a heritable translocated chromosome which can be identified in mitotic cells. This mouse is called CBA/T6T6. CBA mice were irradiated and repopulated with CBA thymus cells and CBA/T6T6 bone marrow cells. The antibody-forming cells were then examined for the presence of the T6T6 chromosome marker. The antibody-producing cells contained the marker showing that the bone marrow-derived cells produced the antibody. When the experiment was carried out in the other direction, i.e., with thymus cells which had the marker and bone marrow cells which did not, none of the antibody-forming cells contained the T6T6 marker.

This shows that it is the bone marrow-derived cells which produce antibody and thus are the effector cells in antibody formation and that it is the cells of the thymus which act as helper cells since the bone marrow cells alone cannot produce antibody. It is also safe to conclude that in the thymectomy experiments in Figure 4, the cells of the thymectomized animal which were producing antibody were the bone marrow-derived lymphocytes. But one should keep in mind the problem that allogeneic thymus cells can reconstitute a neonatally thymectomized mouse, but allogeneic bone marrow and thymus cells cannot cooperate in reconstituting an irradiated host. This problem has not really been successfully addressed even today but will be discussed further in Chapter 9.

T-CELLS AND B-CELLS

We have seen so far that the two primary lymphoid organs are the thymus and the bone marrow (which is probably the mammalian bursal equivalent). We have also seen that thymus-derived lymphocytes have a helper function in the antibody response and that bone marrow-derived lymphocytes are the cells which produce antibody. Current terminology refers to the cells of thymic origin which are in the secondary lymphoid organs as T-CELLS. The lymphocytes in the thymus are referred to as thymocytes or thymic lymphocytes. The cells of bone marrow origin which are able to synthesize antibody are referred to as B-CELLS. The designation "B" can stand for bursal-derived or bone marrow-derived (or simply marrow-derived) interchangeably. Modern immunobiology is the study of the nature, function and interaction of B-cells and T-cells. In the rest of this text we will refer constantly to B-cells and T-cells and urge that the definitions outlined above be kept in mind.

ADHERENT AND NONADHERENT CELLS

From all the above we see that the lymphocytes which are involved in antibody formation are derived from the thymus and the bone marrow; however, another cell type, the *macrophage,* is also important in immune responses. The importance of this *nonlymphoid cell* had been suspected from years of study of *in vivo* antibody responses, but it was not until the invention of *in vitro* methods of generating antibody-forming cells that more precise experiments could be carried out. Once more we see an important advance made independently by two groups on separate continents. Mishell and Dutton in La Jolla, California, and Marbrook in Melbourne devised tissue culture methods for generating *in vitro* primary antibody responses in 1966. These methods have been of crucial importance in all aspects of immunobiology. One of the first questions asked using the new techniques concerned the role of the macrophage in generating antibody response.

Cells of the mouse spleen can be separated into two functional

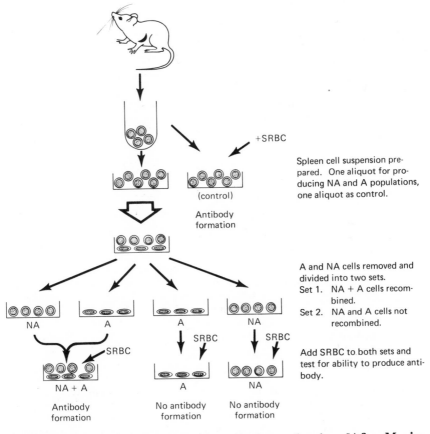

+SRBC

Spleen cell suspension prepared. One aliquot for producing NA and A populations, one aliquot as control.

(control)

Antibody formation

A and NA cells removed and divided into two sets.
Set 1.   NA + A cells recombined.
Set 2.   NA and A cells not recombined.

NA   A   A   NA

SRBC

SRBC   SRBC

NA + A   A   NA

Antibody formation

No antibody formation

No antibody formation

Add SRBC to both sets and test for ability to produce antibody.

5

Nonadherent and adherent cells in antibody production. [**After Mosier (1967).** *Science,* **158, 1573.**]

populations by their differential ability to adhere to the surface of glass or plastic Petri dishes. After a few hours the cells which are not firmly attached to the surface are removed. These are called NONADHERING (NA) cells. The remaining cells are called the ADHERING (A) cells.[4] The NA cells are predominantly lymphocytes, and the A cells are predominantly macrophages. When antigen was added to either the NA or the A cells cultivated *in vitro,* no antibody-forming cells were generated. However, when the adhering and the nonadhering populations were recombined, antibody was produced. This experiment, diagrammed in Figure 5, shows that spleen cells are able to be further divided into two populations, one which contains lymphocytes and one which contains macrophages. These two populations cooperate in generating antibody-forming cells. The role of the macrophage will be discussed in detail in Chapter 11.

THREE CELLS REQUIRED FOR ANTIBODY FORMATION

From these experiments we arrive at what are currently thought to be the cellular components for cell cooperation in antibody formation. The B-cell is the effector cell which synthesizes and secretes antibody. For most antigens the T-cells acts as a helper cell. The process, however, requires the presence of a third, nonlymphocyte, cell, the macrophage.

SUMMARY

1. Removal of the thymus shortly after birth (neonatal thymectomy) abolishes the ability of the animal to generate an antibody response or reject skin grafts. Injection of thymus cells into these animals restores their immune function.

2. Removal of the bursa of Fabricius of the chick early in life abolishes the ability of the animal to generate an antibody response, but the ability to reject skin grafts remains intact. The mammalian equivalent of the bursa is not identifiable, but the bone marrow seems to carry out the function in the mouse.

3. Repopulating lethally irradiated animals with either thymus cells or bone marrow cells alone does not restore the animals' ability to generate antibody responses. Injections of both bone marrow and thymus cells, however, fully restore this capability. This shows that there is cellular cooperation between bone marrow-derived and thymus-derived lymphocyte populations.

[4]Mosier refers to the unattached cells as LYMPHOCYTE RICH (LR) and the attached cells as MACROPHAGE RICH (MR). The terms ADHERING and NONADHERING have come into more common use and will be used in the text.

4. Experiments with cells with surface markers showed that the thymus cells which reconstitute the ability to generate an antibody response in neonatally thymectomized mice are not the cells producing antibody. The reconstituting thymus cells act as helper cells to a cell already present in the animal.

5. Experiments with chromosome markers showed that in bone marrow–thymus reconstitution experiments it is the bone marrow cells which produce the antibody.

6. In antibody formation the bone marrow-derived lymphocyte is the effector cell and the thymus-derived lymphocyte is the helper cell.

7. Bone marrow-derived lymphocytes are called B-cells, and thymus-derived lymphocytes are called T-cells.

8. Removal of macrophages from a spleen cell population takes away the ability of the cells to generate an antibody response.

9. Three cell types interact in antibody formation: B-cells are effector cells which produce antibody, T-cells act as helper cells, and macrophages also participate.

READINGS

Claman, H. N., Chaperon, E. A., and Triplett, R. F. (1966). Thymus-marrow cell combinations. Synergism in antibody production, *Proc. Soc. Exp. Biol. Med.* **122,** 1167. (A paper which convinced many people that cooperation was crucial in generating antibody responses.)

Davies, A. J. S., *et. al.* (1964). The failure of thymus-derived cells to produce antibody, *Transplantation,* **5,** 222. (The suggestion that the thymus cell is not the antibody-producing cell.)

Good, R. A., and Gabrielson, A. E. (ed.) (1964). *The Thymus in Immunobiology,* New York, Harper and Row. (A book which captures the flavor of the excitement of the early 1960s when the roles of the thymus and bursa were first being elucidated.)

Miller, J. F. A. P., Marshall, A. H. E., and White, R. G. (1962). The immunological significance of the thymus, *Adv. Immunol.* **2,** 111. (Early views of Miller.)

Miller, J. F. A. P. and Mitchell, G. F. (1968). Immunological activity of thymus and thoracic duct lymphocytes, *Proc. Nat. Acad. Sci. U.S.A.* **59,** 296. (The paper which shows that a host cell makes antibody in thymus-reconstituted neonatal thymectomized mice.)

Mosier, D. E., (1967). A requirement for two cell types for antibody formation *in vitro, Science,* **158,** 1573. (The need for adherent cells is shown in this paper.)

4

CELL INTERACTIONS IN
CELL-MEDIATED RESPONSES

OVERVIEW

In the previous chapter we began developing the evidence that there are separate lymphocyte populations involved in antibody formation and cell-mediated responses. It will be recalled that neonatal thymectomy abolished both antibody formation and graft rejection (a form of cell-mediated response) but that bursectomy abolished only antibody formation, leaving the graft rejection mechanism intact. We then saw that in antibody formation the bursa-derived lymphocytes (the B-cells) are the effector cells, i.e., the cells which produce antibody. On the other hand, the thymus-derived lymphocytes act as "helper" cells. In this chapter we will show that a similar effector-helper cell relationship is found in cell-mediated responses. In these responses both the effector and helper cells are T-cells.

CELL-MEDIATED RESPONSES DEFINED

Before any evidence about cell-mediated responses can be presented, it is essential to understand the nature of these reactions. The designation cell-mediated responses is used to distinguish those reactions from immune reactions in which antibody is involved. As will be seen below, many cell-mediated responses involve tissue destruction. There are other tissue-destroying reactions, called immediate hypersensitivity reactions, in which antibody plays a central role. Immediate hypersensitivity reactions can be transferred to a normal animal with serum from an immune (or hypersensitive) animal. This is not the case with cell-mediated responses which can be transferred only to a normal animal with the lymphoid cells of a sensitized animal. This means that the product of the B-cell is responsible for immediate hypersensitivity reactions. We will see below that T-cells are responsible for cell-mediated reactions.

Delayed-Type Hypersensitivity (DTH)

This is the traditional form of a cell-mediated response and is best exemplified by the *tuberculin test*. If an individual has come in contact with *Mycobacterium tuberculosis,* the agent which causes tuberculosis, that individual has probably been *sensitized* to the antigens on the organism, meaning that there has been an immune response to the bacterium. We know that the immune response can be humoral (giving rise to antibodies) or cellular (giving rise to sensitized cells). To test for the presence of sensitized cells, a small amount of antigen is injected into the skin. If there are sensitized cells in the individual, these cells will accumulate and cause other cells to be attracted to the site of the injected material. This results in a visible, palpable lump 48 hr after injection. Antibody-mediated skin reactions appear before 24 hr (hence the designation *immediate hypersensitivity*). In experimental animals the DTH reaction cannot be transferred to normal animals by serum (which contains antibody) but only by lymphoid cells.

Allograft Rejection

An ALLOGRAFT is the grafting of tissue from one member of a species to a different member of the same species. For example, grafts from one human to another are allografts. A graft between members of two different strains of mice is also an allograft. If tissues from one strain of mouse are grafted onto another strain, the tissue will begin to grow, but after several days the immune system will cause the graft to stop growing and die. This is called GRAFT REJECTION. This rejection is a cell-mediated phenomenon since it can be transferred to normal animals only with lymphocytes and not with serum.

Graft Versus Host Reaction (GVH)

In the allograft reaction the host is immunologically competent, and the graft, usually skin, does not contain immunologically competent cells so that the host recognizes the antigens of the graft as foreign and responds against them. In such a case the host rejects the graft. In the *graft versus host (GVH) reaction* the roles are reversed. As the name implies, it is the graft which recognizes the antigens of the host and responds against them. This means that the graft in a GVH reaction must contain immunocompetent cells. The GVH reaction is widely used in the laboratory, but, like delayed sensitivity and allograft rejection, it also has clinical implications, especially in bone marrow transplantation. If any immunocompetent lymphocytes have recirculated into the bone marrow, these cells will be transferred with the transplanted bone marrow cells (the graft), and these cells can react against the host. In experimental situations the host is usually rendered immunologically incompetent by either treatment with X-ray or use of very young mice which have not yet acquired full immune competence. These immunologically incompetent hosts are injected with lymphocytes which can react against antigens of the host. The ability to carry out a GVH reaction is limited to cells, and antibody does not play a role.

One of the consequences of a GVH reaction is the enlargement of the spleen of the host. Interestingly, it is primarily the host's own cells which infiltrate and enlarge the spleen although they do this because of the presence of the graft cells reacting against the host. The amount of spleen enlargement, or *splenomegaly,* is taken as a measure of the severity of the GVH reaction. It is expressed as the SPLEEN INDEX, the ratio of the weight of the spleen to the total weight of the animal in the experimental group compared with the same ratio in controls.

$$\text{Spleen index} = \frac{\text{weight of experimental spleen/total body weight}}{\text{weight of control spleen/total body weight}}$$

Control animals in a GVH reaction are recipients which are the same age and sex as the recipients of the experimental group but are injected with cells of the same type as the host, i.e. syngeneic cells. There should be no effect from injecting syngeneic cells into a recipient since the control cells will not recognize the host as foreign and this should give a spleen index of 1.0. By convention a spleen index of 1.3 is considered indicative of a positive GVH reaction.

In carrying out the GVH reaction experimentally, mice of the same age and sex must be used as recipients in both experimental and control groups. Usually these are very young mice (about 1 week old), although adults which have been irradiated are also used. The recipients are usually F_1 in which one of the parents is of the same strain as the cells to be injected. In this manner the host does not recognize the transferred cells as foreign. This procedure is diagrammed in Figure 1. In the diagram, spleen cells of strain A are injected into $(A \times B)$ F_1 hybrids. The A cells (the graft) induce a GVH

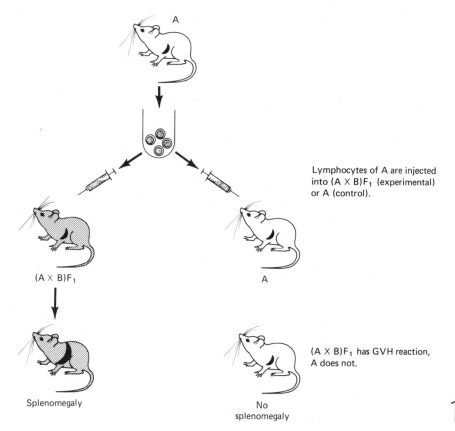

Lymphocytes of A are injected into (A × B)F$_1$ (experimental) or A (control).

(A × B)F$_1$

A

(A × B)F$_1$ has GVH reaction, A does not.

Splenomegaly

No splenomegaly

1

The graft-versus-host reaction.

reaction in (A × B) F$_1$ host but not in the A host. This is because the immunocompetent cells of the A graft recognize the antigens of B on the (A × B) F$_1$ host cells. The cells of the (A × B)F$_1$, however, do not recognize anything as foreign on the A cells. To be sure, the A cells are different since they do not have the B antigens, but immune responses are not made to differences resulting from the absence of antigen, only to the presence of a different antigen. This is diagrammed in Figure 2.

Cell-Mediated Lympholysis (CML)

The two commonly used *in vitro* models of cell-mediated responses are diagrammed in Figure 3. One in which test lymphocytes are lysed

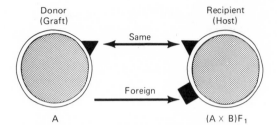

2

The basis of the graft-versus-host reaction. A and (A × B)F share an antigen (▲), but (A × B)F₁ contains an antigen (■) which A lacks. A responds to ■ as foreign. Since A is the graft and (A × B)F₁ is the host, a GVH reaction occurs.

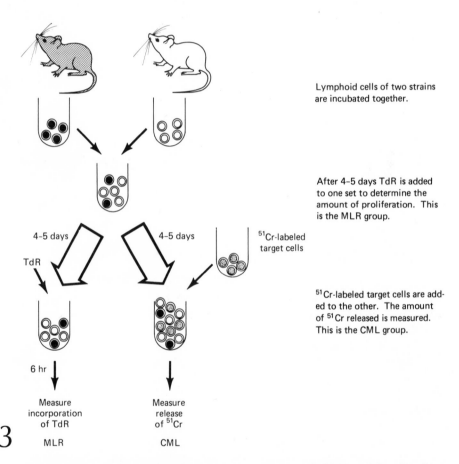

3

Two *in vitro* cell-mediated responses, MLR and CML. [After Bach *et al.*, (1976). *Nature*, **259**, 274.]

in vitro is called CELL-MEDIATED LYMPHOLYSIS (CML). In this reaction cells of one strain of mouse react against antigens on the cells of another strain. Cells of strain A can be injected into strain B so that the strain-B animals are sensitized to A cells (or cells of B can be sensitized to cells of A *in vitro*). In both cases the cells of B are sensitized to A. In the assay to measure the degree of sensitization, the responding cells (in this case cells of strain B) are mixed with *target* cells bearing the relevant antigens A *in vitro*. Target cells bearing A antigens can be cells from strain A or closely related cells which have some of the antigens of A on their surface. These target cells are radiolabeled with radioactive chromium (^{51}Cr). If the radiolabeled target cells are killed by the reaction with the sensitized cells, the chromium label is released into the medium. The amount of released ^{51}Cr is a measure of the amount of target cell lysis, which in turn is a measure of the degree of sensitization.

Mixed Lymphocyte Reactions (MLR)

Another *in vitro* cell-mediated response is called the MIXED LYM-PHOCYTE REACTION (MLR). This reaction measures the amount of cell proliferation which sensitization causes. We will see in Chapter 17 that proliferation is an essential part of the immune response. In the MLR, cells from two individuals or strains which have different surface antigens are mixed together *in vitro*. If one cell population recognizes the other as foreign, it begins to proliferate. This proliferation can be measured by the incorporation of radiolabeled precursors into DNA. In practice the cells are allowed to react for 4 to 5 days, and then tritiated thymidine (TdR) is added to the culture. If there has been proliferation, the TdR will be incorporated into DNA. By extracting the DNA and determining the amount of radiolabel incorporated, a measure of the degree of proliferation is obtained. Since both populations will recognize each other and respond by proliferating, one population can be treated with agents which prevent proliferation, such as mitomycin C or X-ray, so that it cannot proliferate but can still stimulate. This is called a ONE-WAY MLR.

CELLS INVOLVED IN CELL-MEDIATED RESPONSES

Reaction of θ-Positive Cells

We will see in Chapter 5 that there are several surface antigens which serve as markers for different populations of lymphocytes. The most commonly used marker to identify a cell as a T-cell is the presence of the theta (θ) antigen on its surface. θ is an antigen which only thymus-derived lymphocytes express on their surfaces so that if a cell is θ positive, it is by definition a thymus-derived lymphocyte. Treating T-cells with anti-θ antiserum plus complement causes them to lyse. So if cells which can carry out some cell-mediated response are treated with anti-θ plus complement and then lose the ability to carry out the reaction, this is evidence that the cell had θ on its surface and was a thymus-derived lymphocyte.

Figure 4 contains some summarized data showing that the GVH reaction, CML, and MLR are all carried out by θ-positive cells. In each of these experiments the appropriate reaction was carried out with cells which had been treated with normal serum as controls and with a population of cells which were treated with anti-θ and complement. In all cases the anti-θ and complement treatment abolished the cell-mediated response. This is the strongest evidence that cell-mediated responses are carried out by T-cells.

Varied Nature of Cell-Mediated Responses

Delayed hypersensitivity is one of the oldest known reactions in immunology. When allograft rejection came to be investigated as a means of studying skin and organ transplantation, it was soon realized that allograft and delayed hypersensitivity reactions were similar since both were cell-mediated responses. With the discovery that the GVH reaction was a form of rejection phenomenon, it made sense to unify all the cell-mediated reactions and think of them as being roughly equivalent. When *in vitro* reactions such as CML and MLR were found to be cell-mediated reactions, there was initial jubilation because more precise and quantitative means of measuring cell-mediated responses were thought to be available. But as with most initial unifying notions in science, more and more exceptions were found until it became clear that all cell-mediated responses were not merely different manifestations of the same phenomenon measured in different ways. In fact, the various cell-mediated reactions each measure a separate effector or helper T-cell function.

Just as the rapid advances in helper and effector cell cooperation in antibody formation came to dominate so much of immunological thought in the 1960s, helper and effector cell cooperation in cell-mediated responses has come to dominate much thought in the 1970s. It now is becoming quite clear that the different cell-mediated responses are measuring different aspects of T-cell function and also that different subpopulations of T-cells carry out different reactions. In what appears to be developing as a very close analogy to B:T cooperation in antibody formation in which there is an effector and a helper cell, it now is clear that there is T:T cooperation in cell-

Reaction	Stimulator cell	Responder cell	Reaction	Effect of anti-θ treatment of responder cell		
				Normal serum	Anti-θ	Percent reduction
MLR	Balb/c (X-irradiated)	B10	Proliferation as incorp. of TdR (cpm)	8,249	331	94
CML	Balb/c (mitomycin treated)	CBA	Release of ^{51}Cr percent lysis	100	4	96
GVH	CBA	CBA × C57BL/6	Spleen index	1.32	0.91	—

4

Anti-θ treatment abolishes cell-mediated responses. [Data for MLR reaction from Cantor and Boyse (1975). *J. Exp. Med.* **141, 1376. Data for GML reaction from Wagner** *et al.* **(1972).** *Cell Immunol.* **4, 139. Data for GVH reaction from Golub (1971).** *Cell. Immunol.* **2, 353.]**

mediated responses in which one T-cell acts as effector cell and another as helper cell.

CELL COOPERATION IN CELL-MEDIATED RESPONSES

The basic experimental design used in showing that there is cell cooperation in cell-mediated responses is similar in principle to those used in demonstrating cooperation in antibody formation, namely, looking for synergistic effects when cell populations are mixed together. The principle is simple: if one cell population, e.g., thymus, gives X amount of response in the reaction being studied, and a second cell population, e.g., lymph node, also gives X amount of response, then one would predict that thymus *plus* lymph node would give 2X response if they act independently of each other. This would be an ADDITIVE response in which the result is the sum of the two reactions. If the mixture gives a reaction greater than an additive effect, i.e., greater than 2X, then this is a SYNERGISTIC effect and indicates that the two populations are interacting in some way to give an augmented response. In such a case the result of the reaction is greater than the sum of its parts. In all the experiments which follow the hallmark of cell cooperation is a synergistic or greater-than-additive response.

Evidence for Cell Cooperation in GVH Reactions

Cell cooperation in cell-mediated responses was first shown in 1970 by Cantor and Asofsky in the GVH reaction. Using parental thymus cells and peripheral blood cells, they showed that injection of mixtures of cells from these two sites into F_1 hosts resulted in a spleen index in a GVH reaction which was greater than the sum of the two reactions of each of the cell types alone. This important experiment is diagrammed in Figure 5. The recipients were newborn (BALB/c $\times$ C57BL/6)F_1 mice. Varying numbers of parental thymus *or* peripheral blood cells were injected into the F_1, and the spleen index for each concentration of injected cells was noted. A third group of F_1 recipients was injected with both thymus cells *and* peripheral blood cells. The important point in the presentation of the data (Figure 5) is that by varying the number of cells injected, a titration curve relating the spleen index resulting from a certain number of injected cells can be obtained. From this titration curve the number of thymus or peripheral blood cells required to give a positive spleen index of 1.3 can easily be determined. In the experiment in Figure 5 an index of 1.3 was achieved with 5×10^6 thymus cells or with 2×10^5 peripheral blood cells. When thymus and peripheral blood cells are injected together, a synergistic reaction occurs. This is seen from the fact that mixing 5×10^6 thymus with as few as 3×10^4 peripheral blood cells gives an index *greater* than 1.3. Since it takes 2×10^5 peripheral blood lymphocytes to give an index of 1.3, this shows that the thymus cells and peripheral blood cells together are over *10 times* more effective than they would be if the response were additive.

We already saw that the effector cells in GVH reactions are sensitive to anti-θ. When either the thymus cell population or the peripheral blood population in the above experiment was treated with anti-θ, the synergy was abolished, which indicates that both populations are T-cells. Here we have a clear case of T:T interaction.

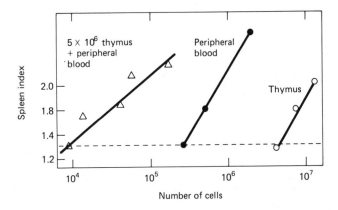

5

Titration curves of cell populations alone or combined in generating a
GVH reaction. The mixture is over 100 times more effective than the
separate populations. [After Asofsky, Cantor and Tigelaar (1971).
Progr. Immunol. **1**, 369.]

Evidence for Cell Cooperation in CML

In the experiments which show that the cells involved in cell-
mediated reactions were T-cells, it was necessary to have a marker (θ)
which distinguished T-cells from B-cells. In the experiments below
which show T:T interaction in CML, it was necessary to have a
marker which distinguished different subpopulations of T-cells. Such
antigenic markers exist as a series of surface antigens called LY
ANTIGENS. These antigens are discussed in detail in Chapter 5. There
are three well-studied Ly antigens termed Ly 1, Ly 2, and Ly 3. In the
experiments which indicate that there are different populations of
T-cells interacting in cell-mediated responses, it was shown that the
interacting populations in another cell-mediated response, CML, had
different Ly antigens on their surfaces.

In the experiment in Figure 6 lymph node T-cells were used to
generate cytotoxic T-cells (i.e., a CML response) *in vitro*. Treatment of
these cells with anti-Ly 1 and complement eliminates all cells which
express Ly 1 on their surface but leaves cells expressing Ly 2 and Ly
3. Similarly, treating the population with anti-Ly 2 and Ly 3 eliminates Ly 2, 3 cells and leaves Ly 1 cells. When Ly 1 T-cells were used
to generate the CML, it was found that they were incapable of
generating a response. Similarly when Ly 2^+, 3^+ cells were used, they
were able to carry out CML at only 30 percent of the control value.
However, when the Ly 1^+ population and the Ly 2^+ population were
mixed, they were able to generate CML at control levels. This shows

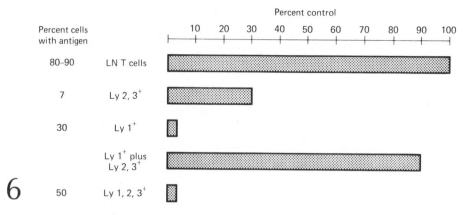

6

Cell cooperation in CML. [After Cantor and Boyse (1975). *J. Exp. Med.* **141, 1376 and 1390.]**

that there are two populations of T-lymphocytes which interact synergistically in CML responses. One of these is the effector cell, but it needs the helper cell to fully generate its cytotoxic capacity. To determine which T-cell is the helper cell and which T-cell is the effector, the following experiment was carried out. A CML was generated with lymph node T-cells, but before the cells were assayed for their ability to cause ^{51}Cr release, they were treated with either anti-Ly 1 or anti-Ly 2, 3. The cells remaining after this treatment were then tested for their ability to act as effector cells in CML. Only treatment with anti-Ly 2 or 3 abolished the ability of the cells to carry out lysis of the target cells. This shows that the Ly 2^+, 3^+ cells are effector cells and the Ly 1^+ cells act as helper cells in CML reactions.

Helper T-cells and Effector T-cells

What this chapter has demonstrated is that there is an analogy between antibody formation and cell-mediated responses. In both kinds of reaction we see one lymphocyte population functioning as an effector population and one as a helper population. In succeeding chapters we will show that the helper cells in both antibody formation and cell-mediated responses react with different antigenic determinants than do the effector cells. This response to different antigenic determinants by the helper-cell population results in an amplification of the helper-cell population which then somehow augments the effector-cell population.

SUMMARY

1. Cell-mediated responses are responses carried out by cells in which anti-body is not involved.
2. The commonly studied forms of cell-mediated responses are delayed-type hypersensitivity (DTH), allograft rejection, graft-versus-host (GVH) reactions, cell-mediated lympholysis (CML), and mixed lymphocyte reactions (MLR).
3. Cell-mediated responses are mediated by T-cells.
4. There is cell cooperation in cell-mediated responses as shown by the synergistic interaction of T-cells from different anatomical sites and by use of anti-Ly antiserum.
5. The effector cell in a CML is an Ly 2^+, 3^+ T-cell, and the helper cell is an Ly 1^+ T-cell.

READINGS

TEXT

Bloom, B. R., and Glade, P. R. (1971). *In Vitro Methods in Cell-Mediated Immunity,* New York, Academic Press. (Description of methods used in studying cell-mediated responses.)

ARTICLES

Asofsky, R., Cantor, H., and Tigelaar, R. E. (1971). Cell interactions in the graft-versus-host response, in Amos (ed.), *Prog. Immunol.* **1,** 369. (Early demonstration of cell cooperation in a cell-mediated response.)

Cantor, H., and Boyse, E. A. (1975). Functional subclasses of T lymphocytes bearing different Ly antigens. I. The generation of functionally distinct T-cell subclasses in a differentiative process independent of antigen, *J. Exp. Med.* **141,** 1376.

——— and ——— (1975). Functional subclasses of T lymphocytes bearing different Ly antigens. II. Cooperation between subclasses of Ly^+ cells in the generation of killer activity, *J. Exp. Med.* **141,** 1390.

(Two papers which define T-cell subclasses by their Ly antigens and show cell cooperation in the CML reaction.)

5

PROPERTIES OF B-CELLS AND T-CELLS

OVERVIEW

So far in this section we have seen that the action of hormone-like factors in the primary lymphoid organs converts the lymphoid progenitor cell into either a thymus-derived or a bursal-derived lymphocyte. After export to the secondary lymphoid tissues these cells become functional B-cells or T-cells which interact with antigen and with each other as described in Chapters 3 and 4. In this chapter we will define some of the physical properties of B-cells and T-cells.

SURFACE ALLOANTIGENS AS CELL MARKERS

One of the most distinctive changes that comes about during lymphoid differentiation is the nature of the surface components of the cell. As the cell differentiates, it begins to express new surface components and stops expressing others. Some of the surface components which change with differentiation are antigenic, and these antigens have been termed DIFFERENTIATION ANTIGENS[1] by Old and Boyse, who have pioneered the use of unique cell surface markers in the study of both normal and leukemic lymphocyte functions. The concept of differentiation antigens is an intriguing one since it implies that fundamental

---

[1]The surface components are antigenic only in another strain or another species which does not express the antigen. For this reason mutant and congenic mice which differ from each other in only a single surface antigen are widely used to generate these antibodies. A detailed discussion of many of the kinds of congenic mice is found in Chapter 6.

changes in the life history of a cell are accompanied by unique structures at the cell surface. What functions, if any, these new antigenic structures have is not known, but they do provide a powerful tool for studying the differentiation process. Many of the differentiation antigens are ALLOANTIGENS. Like allotypes (Chapter 13), alloantigens are antigens which one member of the species may possess and another member may not. These antigens segregate as if they were controlled by allelic genes. To produce an alloantiserum, cells of a mouse of one strain are injected into mice of another strain. It will be recalled that CBA antiserum against C57BL/6 was used to determine that the bone marrow-derived cell and not the thymus-derived cell was producing antibody. This is an example of alloantisera raised against alloantigens.

Most of the information which we have about surface properties of T-cells and B-cells comes from work done in the mouse. Because of the availability of inbred, congenic, and mutant strains of mice, it is possible to produce alloantisera against a wide variety of surface components. In the following section we will briefly describe antigens on the surface of T-cells and B-cells. Some are differentiation antigens, most are alloantigens, but all are used to distinguish between the two lymphoid populations.

SURFACE MARKERS OF T-CELLS

Theta (θ), or Thy 1

One of the most extensively studied alloantigens is theta (θ) or Thy 1. The presence of θ on the surface of a cell is used to distinguish thymic-derived and non-thymic-derived lymphocytes. This antigen was first described by Reiff and Allen who, during the course of immunizing C3H mice with AKR thymocytes, found that they could produce an antiserum specific for thymus-derived lymphocytes. The antibody produced in C3H mice reacted with AKR thymus cells but not thymus of C3H. On the other hand the antibody to C3H thymus produced by AKR reacted with the thymocytes of C3H and several other strains but not AKR. These findings show that the antibody is not directed against an antigen common to thymus-derived lymphocytes of all mice but rather against a thymus antigen which some strains have but others do not, i.e., an alloantigen. When many strains of mice were examined, it was found that most of the common strains (for example, BALB/c, CBA, C57BL/6, DBA/2, and B10) reacted with the anti-C3H antiserum. Only a few strains reacted with the anti-AKR. This argues that there are *two alleles* for the expression of the θ antigen. An animal of a given strain has the allelic gene to express θ of the C3H type (called θ C3H, or Thy 1.2) or θ of the AKR type (called θ AKR, or Thy 1.1) on its thymus-derived lymphocytes.

Theta is expressed on about 95 to 98 percent lymphocytes in the thymus and is not expressed by cells in the bone marrow or on immunoglobulin-positive lymphocytes which are B-cells (see below). When the thymocyte is exported from the thymus to the peripheral lymphoid tissues, the θ antigen is still expressed; i.e., the T-cell is θ positive. Because of this fact, the presence of θ on a lymphocyte is used as one of the ultimate criteria for identifying the cell as a thymus-derived lymphocyte.

While θ appears on thymus-derived lymphocytes and not on B-cells, it is not an organ-specific antigen. The antigen appears on neuronal cells in the brain and on epidermal cells and can be found on cultured fibroblasts. Because it appears on both thymus-derived lymphocytes and brain, it has been possible to immunize rabbits with mouse brain and obtain a heteroantiserum which has many of the properties of an allogeneic anti-θ serum. The chemistry of the θ antigen is being worked out, and the antigen appears to be a glycolipid with characteristics of a ganglioside. The brain-associated θ and thymus θ are structurally very similar, although not identical.

When the thymocyte leaves the thymus for the peripheral lymphoid tissue (becomes a T-cell), it still expresses θ on its surface, but the amount of the antigen per cell is decreased. The percentage of θ-positive cells in the various lymphoid organs is shown in Table 1.

Ly antigens

Another extremely useful series of surface markers are the LY ANTIGENS. Just as the presence of θ on the surface of a lymphocyte is used as the hallmark of the cell being thymus-derived, the presence of

TABLE 1.   PERCENT θ-POSITIVE CELLS IN MOUSE LYMPHOID TISSUE

	Balb/c	*CBA*
Blood lymphocytes	70	70
Lymph node	63	72
Spleen	33	32
Peyer's patches	20	25

From Raff and Owen (1971). *Eur. J. Immunol.* **1,** 27.

the various Ly antigens is rapidly becoming the hallmark of various _subpopulations_ of thymic-derived cells. There are three well-studied Ly antigens called Ly 1, Ly 2, and Ly 3. Each of these comprises a genetic locus. There are two alleles for each Ly antigen. Each allele codes for alternative alloantigens which are designated 1 and 2. Thus Ly 1 has two allelic forms, Ly 1.1 and Ly 1.2. Similarly, Ly 2 has two forms, Ly 2.1 and Ly 2.2. All mice have Ly 1, Ly 2, and Ly 3, but the allelic forms will vary between strains. Thus strain X may be Ly 1.1, Ly 2.1, and Ly 3.2 while strain Y may be Ly 1.2, Ly 2.1, and Ly 3.1. The genes specifying Ly 1 are on chromosome 19, and the genes for Ly 2 and Ly 3 are closely linked on chromosome 6.

Almost all the thymocytes and T-cells of an individual mouse express the appropriate allelic forms of the Ly antigens, but each thymus-derived lymphocyte does not express each of the antigens. What has made these antigens so useful is the fact that different functional subpopulations of T-cells express different Ly antigens. We saw in Chapter 4 that there are synergistic interactions between Ly 1 and Ly 2, 3 cells in generation of CML responses. We will see in Chapter 8 that the effector cell in the CML reaction is Ly 2, 3^+ and the helper cell is Ly 1^+.

Thymus Leukemia Antigen

The THYMUS LEUKEMIA (TL) ANTIGEN is an alloantigen controlled by a gene Tla, which is found adjacent to the major histocompatability complex in the mouse (see Chapter 6). TL has at least three alleles termed TL 1, TL 2, and TL 3. The antigen was first discovered on thymic leukemia cells (hence its name), but it also appears on normal thymus cells of certain, but not all, strains of mice. TL is expressed _only on thymocytes_ and not on peripheral T-cells. It is therefore clearly a differentiation antigen. When the progenitor enters the thymus and differentiates into a thymus lymphocyte, it begins to express TL. When the thymic lymphocyte leaves the thymus, it stops expressing the TL antigen. Thus the thymocyte is TL^+ and the T-cell is TL^-.

There is a very interesting phenomenon called ANTIGENIC MODULATION which is seen with TL. If anti-TL antibody in the absence of complement is added to a population of thymocytes _in vitro,_ the TL antigen disappears from the cell surface and the cell becomes TL^-. When these antibody-treated cells are injected into an animal, they begin to express TL again and become TL^+. It was once thought that this was an example of antibody to a surface component of a cell affecting the expression of the gene coding for the product. However it now seems possible that this is an example of the antibody inducing redistribution of antigens in the membrane by capping and pinocytosis (see Chapter 10 for details).

GIX

GIX is an alloantigen which is found on both thymocytes and T-cells of some strains of mice. The T-cells of a GIX-negative strain can be converted to GIX positive by infection with murine leukemia virus, which suggests that the antigen may be coded by virus genes. The antigen also has recently been shown to be expressed on spermatozoa cells.

A summary of T-cell surface properties is seen in Table 2.

Markers on Human T-Cells

Most of the antigens discussed above are alloantigens, i.e., are produced by immunizing one strain of mice with tissues of another. Obviously this cannot be done in humans, and other means of generating antisera for the serological identification of human T-cells must be found. Several procedures have been used. For example, a rabbit anti-human thymus cell serum (absorbed with cells from patients with chronic lymphocytic leukemia, a B-cell leukemia) has had some success in identifying human T-cells. Anti-human brain, similarly absorbed, has also been of some limited value. Human T-cells appear to bind sheep RBC in a nonspecific manner, and the SRBC rosette-forming human cells correlate well with brain-positive cells and ability to be stimulated by T-cell mitogens (see below). Because of the limitations of testing for T-cell function in humans, we have had to rely very heavily upon the analogy of function with mouse T-cells. In a later section we will discuss nonserological

TABLE 2. SURFACE MARKERS OF MOUSE THYMUS-DERIVED LYMPHOCYTES

Antigens	Alleles	Present on
θ or Thy 1	θC3H or Thy 1.2 θAKR or Thy 1.1	Thymus and T-cells
Ly	Ly 1.1 or Ly 1.2 Ly 2.1 or Ly 2.2 Ly 3.1 or Ly 3.2	Thymus and T-cell subpopulations
TL	TL1, TL2, TL3	Thymus of TL^+ strains, some thymic leukemias
GIX		Thymus, T-cells, and MuLV-infected cells

methods which identify T-cells which seem to have better discriminating power for human T-cells.

SURFACE MARKERS OF B-CELLS

In the section above we talked about the lymphoid progenitor migrating from the bone marrow to the HIM in the thymus where it differentiated into a thymocyte (i.e., expressed θ, TL, Ly). A similar phenomenon occurs with B-cells. The difficulty, however, is that, except in the chicken, we do not know where the B-cell HIM is located. In the chicken it is the bursa of Fabricius; in mammals it is probably diffusely distributed throughout the hematopoietic tissue but located primarily in the bone marrow. In fetal mice the liver apparently acts as a B-cell HIM. There are certain characteristic surface features of B-cells which distinguish them from T-cells.

Immunoglobulin

If the hallmark of the T-cell is surface θ antigen, the hallmark of the B-cell is SURFACE IMMUNOGLOBULIN (Ig). When a population of spleen or lymph node lymphocytes is stained with fluorescent anti-Ig, 70 percent of spleen cells and 30 percent of lymph node cells are Ig positive. This means that they have readily measurable quantities of Ig on their surface. There is some controversy about the amount of surface Ig on T-cells (see Chapter 10), but no matter how this controversy is ultimately resolved, the T-cell surface immunoglobulin, if it exists, is significantly more difficult to find than the B-cell surface immunoglobulin.

As seen in Table 3 the Ig on B-cells appears to be of two classes, IgM and IgD, but there is little or no IgG. It is generally, but not universally, assumed that the surface Ig on the B-cell acts as antigen-specific receptor molecules to initiate B-cell activation. If this is the case, it is not known if IgG, IgM, and/or IgD are the receptors. This will be discussed in more detail in Chapter 10.

TABLE 3. PROPORTION OF Ig CLASS ON MOUSE SPLEEN B-LYMPHOCYTES

Class of Ig	Percent cells	Description
IgM	20–30	Large lymphocytes
IgD	30–40 ⎱	
IgM and IgD	40–50 ⎰	Small lymphocytes
IgG	<10	

MBLA

A heteroantiserum, ANTI-MOUSE-SPECIFIC B LYMPHOCYTE ANTIGEN (MBLA), has been generated by immunizing rabbits with lymph node lymphocytes obtained from thymectomized, irradiated, fetal-liver-reconstituted mice. When the antiserum is extensively absorbed with thymocytes, it reacts with B-cells of the bone marrow and spleen, plaque-forming cells, and myeloma cells but not T-cells. MBLA thus appears to be an antigen common to all B-cells.

PC1

PLASMA CELL ANTIGEN (PC1) is an antigen found on antibody-secreting cells and not on B-cell precursors. This antigen is also shared with brain.

Fc and C receptors

In addition to the antigens described above, there are two nonantigenic markers on lymphocytes which are found predominantly on B-cells. Both of these are receptors. One of the receptors on the surface of the B-cells reacts with the Fc portion (see Chapter 13) of antigen-antibody complexes or aggregated Ig and is called the *Fc receptor*. This receptor can be demonstrated by showing that a complex of erythrocyte and antibody (EA) will form rosettes (see Figure 1) or that labeled aggregated Ig will bind to lymphocytes. The binding in both cases is via the Fc portion of the Ig molecule. The binding is to the B-cells since the cells that are positive for the Fc receptor are also Ig positive and θ negative.

B-cells also have a receptor which reacts with antigen-antibody-complement complexes. This is called the *complement receptor*. If erythrocytes are reacted with anti-erythrocyte antibody, an antigen-antibody complex is formed. If complement is now added in such a manner that lysis of the erythrocytes does not occur, an antigen-antibody-complement complex (EAC) is formed. This EAC, when reacted with lymphocytes, forms rosettes (see Figure 1). The rosette is formed through the interaction of the complement part of the EAC with a receptor for complement on the lymphocyte. Lymphocytes which form EAC rosettes are called COMPLEMENT RECEPTOR LYMPHOCYTES (CRL). Only complement which has reacted with the antigen-antibody complex will work; i.e., complement in the absence of the antigen-antibody complex will not bind. The component of complement which is involved is a split product of C3. CRL are B-cells since they are θ negative, their proportions increase after neonatal thymectomy, and they have surface Ig.

A summary of surface properties of B-cells is presented in Table 4.

Formation of EA and EAC rosettes to detect Fc and C receptors on lymphocytes.

ANTIGENS ON BOTH B- AND T-CELLS

Ia Antigens

In the next chapter (Chapter 6) we will discuss H-2, the major histocompatability complex, in great detail. However, one portion of the H-2 complex, called the I region, must be discussed here. It is

TABLE 4.   SUMMARY OF SURFACE PROPERTIES OF B-CELLS

Immunoglobulin   (Ig)
Mouse-specific B lymphocyte antigen   (MBLA)
Plasma cell antigen   (PC1)
Fc receptor
C receptor

possible to generate alloantisera presumably directed against products of the I region of the H-2 gene complex. Some *but not all* of these Ia (I-associated) antigens may be specific B-cell markers. The presence of Ia on activated thymus-derived cells has been known for several years. ConA-activated T-cells, for example, are Ia positive.

Very recent data has shown that the suppressor T-cell (Chapter 18) is Ia^+. This is important because both the suppressor T-cell and the cytotoxic T-cell in a CML are Ly 2, 3^+. The fact that the suppressor cell is Ia^+ but the cytotoxic cell is Ia^- shows that they are different cells.

Null Cells

A small population of cells are both θ and Ig negative. These have been termed NULL CELLS. It is not clear at the present time what the significance of this population may be. There are cells called NATURAL KILLER (NK) CELLS which have cytolytic activity against tumors. The null cells may be a subpopulation of the NK cells.

PROLIFERATIVE RESPONSES OF T- AND B-CELLS

Mitogenic Stimulation of Lymphocytes

Up to now we have been discussing surface properties of lymphocytes. Another commonly used and extremely valuable means of distinguishing B-cells from T-cells is by their differential responses to various substances which induce proliferation. These substances are called MITOGENS. A mitogen is a substance which induces a cell into mitosis. Since mitosis involves the production of new DNA, the amount of mitosis which a cell population is undergoing can be quantitated by measuring the amount of DNA synthesized. Since mitosis correlates strongly with proliferation, a reasonable measure of proliferation is obtained by measuring the amount of DNA synthesized. This is done by measuring the amount of radiolabeled DNA precursor (usually tritiated thymidine, ^3H) incorporated into DNA. The tritiated thymidine is added to cultures for short periods of time, and the amount of label incorporated into DNA is measured. This process is seen diagrammatically in Figure 2.

It had been observed in the early 1960s that some lectins isolated from plants induced blast cell transformation in lymphocyte populations. Blast cells are large, metabolically active, lymphocytes, and their presence is an indication of intense cellular activity. A close correlation was found between the amount of blastogenesis (blast cells formed after treatment) and incorporation of tritiated thymidine

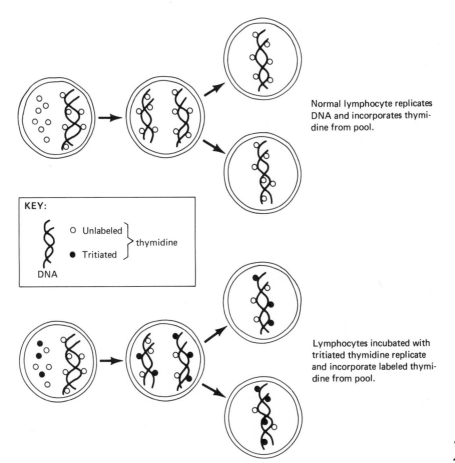

Normal lymphocyte replicates DNA and incorporates thymidine from pool.

KEY:

○ Unlabeled
● Tritiated } thymidine

DNA

Lymphocytes incubated with tritiated thymidine replicate and incorporate labeled thymidine from pool.

2

Incorporation of tritiated thymidine into DNA as a measure of cell proliferation.

into DNA. Because the incorporation of radiolabel is an easier and better quantitative method than the microscopic examination of stained preparations, it is now the almost universally used method for determining if a substance is mitogenic.

Some of the most commonly used mitogens are: PHYTOHEMAGGLUTININ (PHA), CONCANAVALIN A (Con A), POKEWEED MITOGEN (PWM), and BACTERIAL LIPOPOLYSACCHARIDE (LPS). All these (and many more) substances, when added to cultures of either spleen, lymph node, thymus, or peripheral blood, induce intense mitogenic activity. A typical mitogenicity experiment is illustrated in Figure 3.

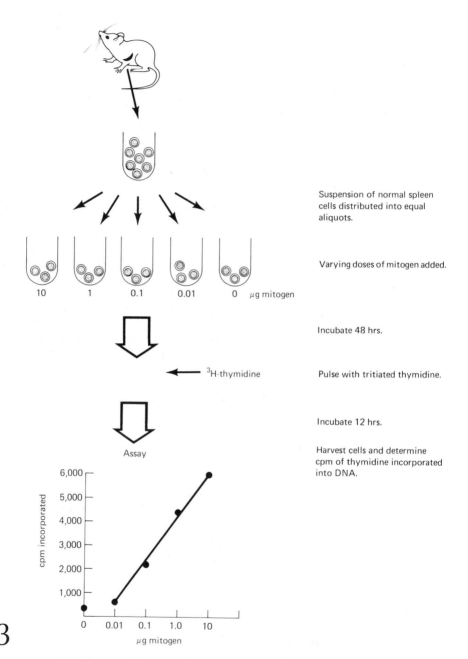

Suspension of normal spleen cells distributed into equal aliquots.

Varying doses of mitogen added.

Incubate 48 hrs.

Pulse with tritiated thymidine.

Incubate 12 hrs.

Harvest cells and determine cpm of thymidine incorporated into DNA.

3

A typical mitogen experiment.

Mitogen Responses of B- and T-Cells

With the growing awareness that B-cells and T-cells were so very different in their functions and surface properties, it was natural to determine if both types of lymphocytes were equally stimulated by the commonly used mitogens.

To examine the effect of various mitogens on B-cells and T-cells, Jannosy and Greaves carried out the following very important experiment. The adherent cells (macrophages) were removed from a normal spleen cell population, and the nonadherent cells (lymphocytes) were treated with anti-θ and complement to remove T-cells. This left a "B-spleen," a population of spleen cells extremely enriched in B-cells and with very few T-cells or macrophages. This allowed the investigators to study mitogen responses of the B-cells in the virtual absence of T-cells and macrophages. These "B-spleen" cells were then cultured in the presence of PHA, ConA, or PWM, and the amount of tritiated thymidine incorporated into DNA was determined. The results in Figure 4 show that PHA and ConA did not stimulate the cells but PWM was a potent mitogen for B-cells. The experiment also shows that ConA stimulates thymocytes but that PHA does not. However, both PHA and ConA stimulate *cortisone-resistant thymocytes*. It will be seen below that cortisone-resistant thymocytes function in all respects like functional T-cells of the peripheral or secondary lymphoid tissue. Taken together, the findings of this experiment show that ConA and PHA act as mitogens for thymus-derived lymphocytes but not for B-cells. PWM (and LPS) act as B-cell mitogens but do not stimulate T-cells.

FUNCTIONAL MATURATION OF THYMIC LYMPHOCYTES

We already know that the lymphoid progenitor cells, upon entering the thymus via the blood (the thymus has no afferent lymphatics), begin to express θ, TL, Ly, and GIX. The lymphocytes which leave the thymus to become T-cells in the peripheral lymphoid organs continue to express θ, Ly, and GIX on their surface but no longer express TL. Thus T-cells are TL(−) even in TL(+) strains of mice. However there is a small population (*ca.* 2 to 5 percent) of thymocytes in the thymus of TL(+) strains of mice which are TL(−). By the criterion of the absence of this differentiation antigen these cells have the characteristics of peripheral thymus-derived cells. It is generally (but, as usual, not universally) thought that these TL⁻ cells are the most mature thymocytes and are ready for export to the peripheral lymphoid tissues.

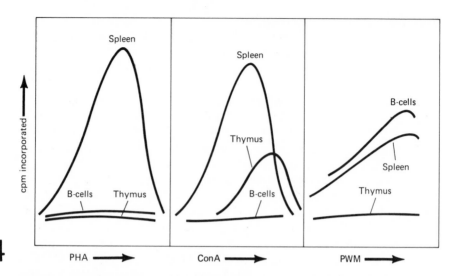

4

Differential responses of lymphocytes to various mitogens. [After Jannosy and Greaves (1972). *Clin. Exp. Immunol.* **10, 525.]**

To determine if there is a *functional* difference between the TL⁺ and TL⁻ thymus lymphocytes, the GVH-inducing capacity of the total thymus lymphocyte population and only the TL⁻ fraction were compared with lymph node T-cells which are all TL⁻. Recall that the GVH reaction is carried out by T-cells (Chapter 4) and that lymph node cells are approximately 70 times better at initiating GVH reactions than are thymus cells. Approximately 95 percent of thymus cells are TL⁺, and only 5 percent are TL⁻, but lymph node T-cells are all TL⁻. When the total thymus cell population was compared with the TL⁻ fraction of thymus cells, it was found that 2×10^6 TL⁻ thymocytes had GVH-inducing capacity equal to 15×10^6 total thymus cells (Table 5). Since over 90 percent of the thymus cells are TL⁺, this argues that the cells in the thymus which carry out the function are the TL⁻ cells. Peripheral T-cells are TL⁻, and they have great capacity to carry out GVH reactions, so this experiment shows the functional similarity between the TL⁻ thymocyte and the peripheral T-cell.

Cortisone Sensitivity of Thymus Cells

When mice are injected with hydrocortisone (approximately 2.5 mg per mouse), the quantity of cells found in the thymus is reduced to as little as 10 percent. The remaining cells, those which are resistant

TABLE 5.   COMPARISON OF ABILITY OF TL$^+$ AND TL$^-$ THYMOCYTES TO GENERATE GVH RESPONSES

Cells	Antiserum + complement	Number of cells injected*	Spleen Index 1.0	2.0	3.0
Thymocytes (TL$^+$ & TL$^-$)	none	5×10^6	⋮⋰		
Thymocytes (TL$^+$ & TL$^-$)	none	15×10^6		•	••••
Thymocytes (TL$^-$)	anti-TL	2×10^6		•••	•••
Lymph node (TL$^-$)	none	2×10^5			••••••

*(BALB/c $\times$ C57BL/6)F$_1$ neonates were injected with C57BL/6 cells as indicated. Data from Leckband and Boyse (1971). *Science* **172**, 1258.

to cortisone treatment, are found to be TL$^-$. Since we already know that the TL$^-$ cells are functional in GVH reactions, it was natural to determine if the cortisone-resistant thymus (CRT) cells are also functional; experiments to settle this point were carried out simultaneously in several laboratories around the world. The results showed very clearly that cortisone-resistant thymocytes are capable of GVH and helper activity. We already saw (Figure 4) that thymocytes respond poorly to PHA but that CRT cells make good responses to this mitogen.

Functional Maturation of Thymus-Derived Cells
   This data argues that the cortisone-resistant thymocyte shares characteristics with peripheral T-cells and is used in the argument that there is *functional maturation* of lymphocytes in the thymus. The maturational scheme is thought to be one of progenitor cell to immature thymocyte to "mature" thymocyte. The "mature" thymocyte is "exported" to the peripheral tissues as a functional T-cell. These properties are summarized in Table 6.

Thymus-Dependent Areas
   The "mature" cells which leave the thymus become localized in specific areas of the secondary lymphoid tissue. The experiments

TABLE 6.   SUMMARY OF PROPERTIES OF "IMMATURE" AND "MATURE"
THYMOCYTES AND PERIPHERAL T-CELLS

Property	"Immature" thymocyte	"Mature" thymocyte	Peripheral T-cells
Surface antigens	TL, θ, Ly	θ, Ly	θ, Ly
Cortisone sensitivity	Sensitive	Resistant	Resistant
T-cell function	No	Yes	Yes
Location in thymus	Cortex	Medulla	(Exported)

which identified these areas were carried out by examining the
spleens and lymph nodes of neonatally thymectomized mice before
and after repopulation with labeled syngeneic thymus or spleen cells.
Neonatally thymectomized mice were injected with thymus or spleen
cells which were labeled *in vitro* with tritiated adenosine, and the
fate of the cells followed by autoradiography. In the spleens of the
neonatally thymectomized mice before repopulation there were areas
depleted of lymphocytes. When the thymectomized animals were
repopulated with labeled thymus cells, these areas became repopulated with labeled cells. These areas are called the THYMUS-DEPENDENT
AREAS of the spleen and lymph nodes.

SUMMARY

1. T-cells can be identified by unique surface alloantigens. The most useful
   are θ (Thy 1), Ly, and TL. Some of these are differentiation antigens.
2. Lymphocytes in the thymus express θ, Ly, and TL. Thymus-derived
   lymphocytes in the secondary lymphoid tissue express θ and Ly but not
   TL. Functional subpopulations bear different Ly antigens.
3. B-cells are characterized by large amounts of Ig on their surfaces. They
   also have receptors for complement and Fc.
4. Thymus-derived cells are induced into mitosis by the mitogens PHA and
   ConA. B-cells are induced into mitosis by PWM and the mitogen LPS.
5. A minority subpopulation of thymus cells are TL$^-$ and cortisone resistant.
   These cells have immune functions similar to T-cells in the periphery. It is
   thought that they are mature thymocytes ready to be exported to the
   periphery.
6. Thymus cells exported to peripheral lymphoid organs are located in areas
   of the spleen and lymph nodes called thymus-dependent areas.

READINGS

BOOK

Greaves, M. F., Owen, J. J. T., and Raff, M. C. (1974). *T and B Lymphocytes,* New York, American Elsevier. (A complete compilation of facts and ideas about the nature of T and B cells.)

REVIEWS

Boyse, E. A., and Old, L. J. (1969). Some aspects of normal and abnormal surface genetics, *Ann. Rev. Genet.* **3,** 269. (The notion of differentiation antigens is developed in this review.)

Boyse, E. A., Old, L. J., and Stockert, E. (1965). The TL (thymus leukemia) antigen: A review, in *IV International Symposium on Immunopathology,* P. Grabar and P. A. Miescher (eds.), Basel, Schwabe and Co., 23.

Golub, E. S. (1971). Brain-associated θ antigen: Reactivity of rabbit anti-mouse brain with mouse lymphoid cells, *Cell. Immunol.* **2,** 353. (An alternative way of generating anti-θ antiserum and examples of testing the effect of the antiserum on T-cell functions.)

Jannosy, G., and Greaves, M. F. (1972). Lymphocyte activation. I. Response of T and B lymphocytes to phytomitogens, *Clin. Exp. Immunol.* **9,** 483. (Differential responses of T and B cells to mitogens.)

Möller, G. (ed.) (1971). *Surface Antigens on Nucleated Cells, Transplant. Rev.* Vol. 6

———— (1972). *Lymphocyte Activation by Mitogens, Transplant. Rev.* Vol. 11.

———— (1973). *T and B Lymphocytes in Humans. Transplant. Rev.* Vol. 16. (The volumes in this series have articles ranging from reviews to data papers showing differential mitogenic responses of T and B cells in mice and men.)

Raff, M. C. (1970). Two distinct populations of peripheral lymphocytes in mice distinguished by immunofluorescence. *Immunology,* **19,** 637. (The demonstration that θ-negative cells are Ig positive.)

Reif, A. E., and Allen, J. M. V. (1964). The AKR thymic antigen and its distribution in leukemias and nervous tissues, *J. Exp. Med.* **120,** 413. (The first demonstration of θ antigen.)

Stutman, O. (1976.) Two main features of T cell development: Thymus traffic and post thymic maturation, *Contemp. Top. Immunol.,* Vol. 7, in press. (A review of thymocyte and T-cell maturation and a view different from the one developed in this chapter.)

6

THE MAJOR HISTOCOMPATABILITY
COMPLEX: H-2 AND HLA

OVERVIEW

On several occasions in the chapters in this section we have referred
to H-2, the major histocompatability complex (MHC) of the mouse. As
the subject of cell interaction and regulation develops, we will be
referring more and more to phenomena associated with H-2, so it is
important to cover the subject in greater detail at this point.

H-2, the major histocompatability complex of the mouse, is a
complex of multiallelic genes located on one region of chromosome 17.
The genes in this region control a wide variety of surface antigens
and lymphoid functions. This chapter will discuss some of the traits
controlled by the H-2 gene complex and give an overview of the
genetics of the complex. It will be seen that the H-2 complex is a
linked series of genes which control a large variety of immunological
phenomena. Understanding of transplantation, GVH reactions, interaction of B- and T-cells, genetic control of the immune response,
and several other phenomena depend upon understanding the nature
of the H-2 complex. Furthermore, recent discoveries seem to point to
the possibility that H-2 may be crucial in recognition of antigen as
well as in the response to it.

Historical Background

In the 1930s Peter Gorer in England became increasingly dubious
about the then current interpretations and conclusions concerning

transplantation genetics in the mouse. He set himself the very formidable task of reanalyzing the field to answer some of the problems created by the general conclusions of previous work. Gorer began by looking at blood group antigens in the few strains of inbred mice which were available at that time and found two antigen systems. One of these was common to all the strains, differing between them only in quantity. This antigen was designated antigen I. The other antigen was found in some strains but not in others and was called antigen II. Gorer and George Snell of the Jackson Laboratory in Bar Harbor, Maine, showed that the presence of this second antigen correlated with skin graft rejection and tumor immunity. It thus appeared that the second antigen was part of a major histocompatability system of the mouse. It was eventually termed H-2 (H for histocompatability). As work went along, it became very clear that H-2 was a multigene, multiallele complex. With Snell's development of congenic and recombinant strains of mice (see below), analysis of this very complex gene locus became possible.

TRAITS CONTROLLED BY THE GENES OF THE H-2 COMPLEX

Table 1 lists the traits known to be controlled by the genes in the H-2 complex. It is obvious from glancing at the list that there is a dazzling array of traits which seem to bear no relationship to each other. It

TABLE 1. TRAITS CONTROLLED BY GENES
OF THE H-2 COMPLEX

Serologically detected cellular alloantigens
Transplantation antigens
Cell-mediated lympholysis target antigens
Mixed lymphocyte reaction
Immune responses
Graft-versus-host reaction
Serologically defined I antigen (Ia antigens)
T-cell–B-cell interactions
Hybrid resistance
Tumor virus susceptibility
Serum serological protein
Testosterone levels
Complement levels
Liver cyclic adenosine monophosphate levels

After Shreffler and David (1975). *Adv. Immunol.* **20**, 125.

may be comforting to know, however, that as more work is carried out on the H-2 complex, more of the traits become related. After covering some basic H-2 genetics, the rest of this chapter will deal with some of these traits.

GENETICS OF THE H-2 COMPLEX

Mapping the H-2 Complex

The H-2 complex is a linked series of genes in a small segment of chromosome 17. The H-2 map has recently been reordered primarily through the work of Donald Shreffler and Jan Klein. The complex is generally divided into four main REGIONS, K, I, S, and D. The regions are divided into SUBREGIONS.[1] Each region or subregion contains a minimum of one gene called a MARKER GENE which controls a testable trait. The K and D regions of the complex control cellular alloantigens. The I region controls specific immune responses, and the S region controls the quantity of a serum protein which the mouse produces. Each of the genes can therefore be seen to be defined by a product or trait. There are at least six genes in the complex (Figure 1). The I region has at least three subregions, IA, IB, and IC.

The boundaries of the regions and subregions are defined by analysis of *intra-H-2 recombinant mice*. These are mice in which a crossover has occurred within the H-2 complex. The limits of the regions and subregions are always defined by crossovers. If apparently different traits are being studied, only by showing that they may be separated by a crossover event can one determine that the traits are actually controlled by separate genes.

Each of the regions is multiallelic; i.e., each of the genes which defines the region or the subregion appears in one of many forms. The combination of all the alleles at all loci within the complex is called the HAPLOTYPE (see Table 2). The haplotype is denoted with a letter superscript, for example, $H-2^k$ or $H-2^d$. There are reference strains of mice for the standard haplotypes which are called TYPE STRAINS. For example, DBA/2 is the type strain for the $H-2^d$ haplotype; C57BL/10 (called B10) is the type strain for the $H-2^b$ haplotype. Each of the regions of the complex of the strains is designated with a small letter as seen in Table 2.

Strain-A mice are recombinants of $H-2^k$ and $H-2^d$. This strain has

---

[1]There are actually five regions. The most recently defined by crossovers is named G and is discussed later in this chapter. Because this region has not yet worked its way into the general literature, the H-2 complex will be treated as if it had only K, I, S, and D regions. Similarly, we will discuss only three subregions of the I region (IA, IB, IC), even though at least four more subregions have been identified by crossovers.

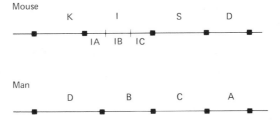

The major histocompatibility complexes of mouse and man. [After Snell, Dausset, and Nathenson (1976). *Histocompatability.*]

the K and I regions of H-2^k and the S and D regions of H-2^d (as seen in Table 2). The K and I regions together are called the K END of the complex, and the S and D regions are called the D END of the complex.

As we stated above, the use of intra-H-2 genetic recombinants with known crossovers is the tool employed to define a region or subregion. By having an assay for a given trait (e.g., an alloantiserum to react with the alloantigen coded for by a gene), one can look for recombinant animals.

Congenic Mice

Another powerful tool is the use of *congenic mice*. If one has two groups of mice which differ at one locus but are the same at all other genetic loci, these animals are called COISOGENIC or CONGENIC. An example would be groups of B10 mice which have different H-2

TABLE 2. H-2 HAPLOTYPES OF SOME COMMONLY USED STRAINS OF MICE AND CONGENICS.

Strain	Haplotype	K	IA	IB	IC	S	D
B10	H-2^b	b	b	b	b	b	b
C57BL/6	H-2^b	b	b	b	b	b	b
DBA/2	H-2^d	d	d	d	d	d	d
BALB/c	H-2^d	d	d	d	d	d	d
C3H	H-2^k	k	k	k	k	k	k
CBA	H-2^k	k	k	k	k	k	k
A	H-2^a	k	k	k	d	d	d
B10.D2	H-2^d	d	d	d	d	d	d
B10.A	H-2^a	k	k	k	d	d	d
B10.BR	H-2^k	k	k	k	k	k	k

haplotypes but identical genes at all other loci (the other loci are called "background" genes).

For example, suppose we wanted to test the role of the H-2 complex on some aspect of the immune response. We would need mice which differ *only* at H-2 and not at any background genes, in other words, mice with the same background genes but different H-2 genes. This would allow us to compare the response of, as an example, B10 mice which are H-2^b with the response of mice with some other H-2 haplotype, say H-2^a. If there were a difference in the response to a certain antigen between the strains, it could be attributed to a difference in H-2 genes and not in background genes. The mice which have B10 background genes and H-2^a genes would be congenic for H-2. If the donor of the H-2^a genes was strain A, the congenic mouse would be designated B10.A. The convention is that the background strain is written first and the donor of the one differing gene or gene complex is written last with a period in between. This notation must not be confused with the designation of an F1 which shows both strains encased in parentheses. For example, an F1 of B10 and A would be (B10 × A).

Production of Congenic Mice

It is obvious that to produce mice which differ at only one specified gene locus requires some fancy genetic footwork. Suppose we have two strains, X and Y. A certain tumor is accepted (will grow) when injected into strain X but will be rejected (will not grow) by strain Y. The object is to introduce the genes of strain Y (the ability to reject this tumor) onto the background of X so that we end up with an X.Y mouse in which the only Y trait is the ability to reject the tumor.

The genetics involved is diagrammed in Figure 2. The procedure involves identifying an animal with the desired trait (the ability to reject the tumor) and backcrossing it to X. This procedure is repeated for several generations. The only trait of Y which is being selected for is ability to reject the tumor, and so the other genes of Y are being diluted at each generation. With each backcross there is further dilution until somewhere around the fifteenth backcross generation the dilution is almost complete, and the result is a strain which has background genes of strain X and graft rejection genes of strain Y.

The example above is a scientific one, but an intuitive example may be of some use. Suppose you decide to systematically determine the amount of vermouth you want in your martinis. You could start by adding to a chilled glass 1 jigger of vermouth, 1 jigger of gin, and an olive. After sipping it, you decide it should be drier, so you discard half of the martini (retaining the olive) and add an equal volume of

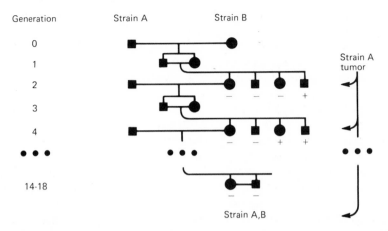

Diagram showing the cross-intercross method of producing congenic resistant lines. Graft acceptance = +, graft rejection = −. [From Snell and Stimpfling (1966). *Biology of the Laboratory Mouse,* **45.]**

gin. Another sip tells you that this is still not dry enough, so you discard half of the martini, retain the olive, and add an equal volume of gin. Another sip, another discard (not the olive, though), and another addition of an equal volume of gin follow. If you do this 10 times you will have a chilled glass which contains over 99 percent gin and the olive. Consider the gin to be the background and the olive to be the desired gene, and you have the notion of a congenic mouse.[2]

K AND D REGIONS

Transplantation Antigens

The H-2 complex is called the major histocompatability complex because of its importance in graft rejection. Until very recently the ultimate test for genetic relatedness between two mice was the rate at which a skin graft from one was rejected by the other. Inbred strains of mice were defined to a large extent by their ability to reject the tissue of another strain. We now know that the antigens which are recognized and reacted against in graft rejection are coded for in the K and D regions of the H-2 complex. If skin of B10 (H-2^b, bbbbbb) is grafted onto DBA/2 (H-2^d, dddddd) and onto C57BL/6 (H-2^b, bbbbbb), it will be rejected in 7 to 10 days by DBA/2 but will grow on C57BL/6 for several weeks before being rejected. B10 and DBA/2 differ at H-2, while B10 and C57BL/6 have the same H-2 haplotype.

[2]I thank Dr. Jan Klein for this instructive illustration.

C57BL/6 will eventually reject the B10 skin because of minor histocompatability antigens (for example, H-1, H-3). This kind of exercise shows that H-2 is the major factor which controls graft rejection. It is the antigens coded in the K and D regions of the complex to which the recipient of the graft responds.

Serologically Defined Antigens

When skin is grafted (or if cells are injected) from mice of one strain to mice of another strain, the recipient strain may also respond by producing antibodies to antigens on the foreign tissue. If the two strains differ at the K and D regions of H-2, then antibody against antigens in these regions will be produced. (Remember that graft rejection is cell mediated, so these antibodies are not responsible for graft rejection.) These antigens are termed the SEROLOGICALLY DEFINED ANTIGENS of the K and D regions. There are many serologically defined antigens which are identified by immunizing one strain with tissues from another strain. The resulting antiserum is then tested for its ability to react with the antigens on cells of a wide variety of strains. Each specificity identified in this manner has been assigned a number. There are now at least 45 known antigenic specificities that are associated with serologically defined antigens in the K and D regions.

A given haplotype has serologically defined antigens unique to that haplotype which are termed PRIVATE SPECIFICITIES. For example, all H-2^k mice have the same serologically defined antigens (numbers 23 and 32). There are many strains of mice with the H-2^k haplotype, and they all contain these private specificity antigens. In addition to the private specificities there are a set of serologically defined antigens which are called PUBLIC SPECIFICITIES. These antigens are not restricted to a given haplotype, and a strain may have several of them while another strain may have some of them as well as others. If the example of H-2^k is used again, animals of strains with the H-2^k haplotype have antigen specificity 3, but this antigen is shared by virtually all haplotypes (for example, H-2^a, H-2^d, H-2^s). Antigen 3 is therefore a public specificity antigen.

It is not resolved whether the serological specificities described above are the specificities involved in graft rejection, i.e., are the major transplantation antigens, although the evidence points in this direction. If these antigens should turn out not to be the transplantation antigens, it would mean that there is another set of antigens coded for in K and D which are not serologically detected but are involved in cell-mediated rejection of foreign tissue.

Cell-Mediated Lympholysis

In Chapter 4 we discussed cell-mediated lympholysis (CML). This is a T-cell mediated reaction which causes the lysis of cells. The antigens on the target cells to which the effector cells in the CML are responding are coded in the K and D regions of H-2. In a later chapter (Chapter 8) we will introduce the notion of serologically defined (SD) and lymphocyte defined (LD) antigens. The antigens coded in the K and D regions of H-2 are the SD antigens. Cells from almost all tissues have serologically defined antigens, although the quantities of these antigens may vary from cells of one organ to those of another.

The mixed lymphocyte and GVH reactions are controlled in part by the K and D region specificities, but the major part of these reactions seems to be coded for in the I region (see below).

Hybrid Resistance

The rules of transplantation say that a graft from a parent should be accepted by an F1 since the F1 (which has the antigens of both parents) should not recognize the parental antigen as foreign. This rule holds in most cases, but transplantation of bone marrow is an exception. In some but not all genetic combinations the F1 hybrid resists the transplanted marrow graft. This intriguing but largely unexplained phenomenon is called HYBRID RESISTANCE. The genes which control this resistance to growth of bone marrow grafts are in a locus called Hh-1 and are associated primarily with the D region of the H-2 complex.

I REGION

The I region codes for several immunologically important traits. This region was discovered only recently and has quickly become of extreme interest.

Immune Response to Specific Antigens

The genetics of the immune response is covered in detail in Chapter 19. In that chapter it will be seen that the ability of mice to make high or low antibody responses to a variety of antigens is correlated with their H-2 haplotypes. Elegant mapping studies using congenic and recombinant mice have localized the gene(s) which control the ability to respond to a wide variety of antigens to the right of K and the left of S. The region is called I for *immune response*.

The I region has at least three multiallelic subregions, all defined by crossovers. These regions are designated I-A, I-B, and I-C, although several new subregions have already been identified.

Susceptibility to Viral Oncogenesis

The susceptibility of mice to the effects of several *tumor viruses* is associated with the H-2 complex and is localized in the I region. This association was initially shown with susceptibility to Gross virus-induced leukemia and has since been shown with Friend virus, radiation leukemia virus (RadLV), mammary tumor virus (MTV) and lymphocytic choriomeningitis virus (LCM). All these could be under the control of one gene, RgV-1 (resistance to Gross virus-1). Susceptibility in all cases is associated with the H-2^k haplotype. It has been suggested that the mechanism of the susceptibility is failure to generate immune responses against the virus.

Stimulation of Mixed Lymphocyte and GVH Reactions

As discussed in Chapter 4, the MLR is a T-cell reaction in which lymphocytes from one strain, when mixed with those of another strain, respond to the allogenic antigens by undergoing proliferation. The extent of proliferation is measured by the incorporation of tritiated thymidine. When the MLR was first discovered, it was thought to be an *in vitro* correlate of histocompatability differences—perhaps even a useful screening procedure for grafting. However, it has become clear that the antigens which are responded against in an MLR are all in the K end (K and I regions) of the H-2 complex since D-end differences (S and D regions) lead to negligible responses. When congenic mice with defined recombinations were tested, it was found that the predominant region of the H-2 which is associated with MLR is the I region. In other words, the strongest MLR were generated when the parties differed in the I region. Other H-2 and non-H-2 differences give only weak stimulation to MLR.

The GVH reaction was also known to be H-2 associated. When the regions of the H-2 complex were analyzed, it was found that as in MLR, differences in the I region are responsible for the major differences leading to the GVH reaction.

These findings have led to the notion of *lymphocyte-activating determinant* genes. It seems that within the I region there are more or stronger lymphocyte-activating determinant genes than in K or D.

B-Cell:T-Cell Interactions

Chapter 9 gives the details of the association of B-cell:T-cell interactions with the H-2 region. It will be seen that the ability of these cells to cooperate in antibody formation may in some manner be controlled by genes in the I region.

Serologically Defined Antigens of the I Region

The I region not only codes for the responses listed above but also for a series of *serologically defined cell surface antigens*. These alloantigens, which are coded by genes in the I region, are termed I-ASSOCIATED or Ia ANTIGENS. After their initial discovery, it appeared that they were antigens which were expressed only on lymphocytes. Indeed, one of these, a B10.A anti-B10.D2 was initially called anti-β because it was thought to be exclusively a B-cell antigen. This now appears not to be a generalized phenomenon since mitogen-activated T-cells and certain effector T-cells have detectable amounts of Ia on their surfaces. Furthermore, while Ia antigens appear to be predominantly on B-cells and certain subpopulations of T-cells, they are also found in varying concentrations on macrophage, spermatozoa, and epidermal cells. They are absent from erythrocytes, brain, liver, and kidney. It has recently been shown that Ia antigens are found in the serum. These molecules seem to have been shed by T-cells, which may explain why most resting T-cells have low amounts of surface Ia.

S REGION

The marker gene for the S region controls the Ss and Slp serum protein traits. The *Ss protein (serum serological)* is an alpha$_2$-beta globulin which is detected serologically by use of a heteroantiserum. Different strains of mice have either high or low concentrations of Ss in their serum. High Ss strains have as much as 20 times the concentration as low Ss strains. The control of the level is by a single autosomal gene with alleles, Ss^h (high) and Ss^l (low). Studies with recombinant haplotypes have located these genes to the right of I and the left of D.

Slp (sex-limited protein) is a globulin which is also detected serologically, but with alloantisera. It is present in some strains but absent in others. The gene which controls its presence or absence is either closely linked to Ss or identical with it. The two alleles of Slp are termed Slp^a and Slp^o. The Slp antigen is androgen dependent. It is found only in Slp^a males and disappears after castration.

The Ss and Slp proteins are associated with or may actually constitute one of the complement components.

G REGION

The most recently located region, the G region, codes for the appearance of an antigen on erythrocytes. This antigen, which is coded by a gene to the right of S and the left of D, is present on red blood cells of strains of mice of haplotype H-2^f, H-2^j, Hp2^p, Hp2^s, and H-2^k. It is not present on H-2^b, H-2^d, and H-2^q.

MAJOR HISTOCOMPATABILITY COMPLEX IN MAN

Man has a major histocompatability complex analogous to the H-2 complex of the mouse, which is termed HLA. The analogy between the MHC of mouse and man is rather striking. HLA has four allelic "series" of antigens which are roughly comparable with the H-2 regions. HLA antigens are found on almost all cells of the body except red blood cells. The regions of the HLA complex are shown in Figure 1. In man the only genes equivalent to the mouse so far discovered are those governing serologically defined products on the cell surface and those governing the responses of lymphocytes in contact with allogenic cells. While no genes exactly comparable with the I region have been identified, there is a definite association between HLA and certain diseases.

POSSIBLE EVOLUTIONARY SIGNIFICANCE

Some scientists have postulated that the evolutionary significance of a polymorphic complex of genes controlling cell surface structures might be in *cell recognition* phenomena. During differentiation of cells and tissues, cells of similar types organize themselves in ordered patterns. This could be done by recognizing similar cell surface moieties. It will be seen in Chapter 10 that recognition of foreign material by the immune system may be linked to recognition of altered self through altered H-2 molecules and that the T-cell receptor may be associated with H-2. There is another gene locus on the same chromosome as H-2 which is multigenic and multiallelic and controls cell surface antigens on early embryos. This locus, called the T-LOCUS, has been postulated to be the embryonic equivalent of H-2 since the antigens coded by it are expressed in early embryonic development when H-2 antigens are not expressed but then cease to be expressed at the time H-2 antigens begin to appear on cell surfaces. It is a real possibility that both H-2 and T products could be acting as molecules by which cells recognize each other.

SUMMARY

1. A wide variety of traits are controlled by a gene complex termed the major histocompatibility complex. In mouse this complex is called H-2, in man it is called HLA.

2. H-2 consists of five distinct regions, K, I, S, G, D. Each region contains a gene which controls a trait. The regions are defined by a recombinational event.

3. K and D regions code for serologically defined H-2 antigens, transplantation antigens, and several other traits.

4. S codes for the level of a serum serological protein.

5. The I region contains at least three subregions and contains the genes which control responses to certain antigens, MLR, and GVH reactions, and B-cell:T-cell interactions, among other traits.

6. Both H-2 and HLA may have evolved as gene loci responsible for cell interaction and recognition.

READINGS

BOOKS AND REVIEWS

Lengerova, A. (1969). *Immunogenetics of Tissue Transplantation,* Amsterdam, North-Holland Publishing Co. (A thorough historical analysis.)

Klein, J. (1975). *Biology of the Mouse Histocompatability-2 Complex,* New York, Springer-Verlag.

Snell, G. D., Dausset, J., and Nathenson, S. (1976). *Histocompatability,* New York, Academic Press.

(These two books are masterful reviews of the major histocompatability complex.)

Shreffler, D. C., and David, C. S. (1975). The H-2 major histocompatability complex and the I immune response region: Genetic variation, function, and organization, *Adv. Immunol.* **20,** 125. (Excellent review of the I region.)

II

MECHANISMS OF CELLULAR COOPERATION IN THE IMMUNE RESPONSE

In the last section we established the basis for the central notion of cellular immunology, which is the interaction of lymphocyte populations and subpopulations. In this section we will now examine the mechanisms by which the cells interact.

In antibody formation the T-cell acts as helper cell and the B-cell acts as effector cell, and in cell-mediated responses the helper T-cell interacts with the effector T-cell. In all immune responses we are seeing a specific response to antigen. Helper cells and effector cells respond to different antigenic determinants on an antigen molecule in both antibody and cell-mediated responses. In antibody formation the T-helper cell (T_H) reacts with the carrier determinants on an antigen molecule, and the B-cell reacts with the hapten determinants. Antibody is produced by the B-cell against the hapten, but unless the T_H has reacted with the carrier determinants of the antigen, no anti-hapten antibody will be produced by the B-cell. Similarly, in cell-mediated responses the T_H reacts with antigens called lymphocyte defined *(LD)* antigens, and the effector T-cell reacts with antigens called serologically defined (SD) antigens. LD antigens are products of the I region of the H-2 complex, and SD antigens are products of the K and D H-2 regions.

Two classes of models have been developed to try to explain B-cell:T-cell cooperation in antibody formation. In both theories T-cells react specifically with carrier determinants, and B-cells react specifically with hapten determinants on the antigen molecule. The theories differ in explaining how the interactions of T-cell and carrier

79

confer help on the B-cell. One set of theories argues that the helper function of T-cells is carried out by soluble products which the T-cell elaborates after specific interaction with antigen. When the B-cell reacts with hapten determinants and the factor elaborated by the T-cell, it becomes a functional effector cell. The nature of the factor is a subject of intense debate. The other model of interaction of T-cells and B-cells postulates that it is through cell contact. Under some experimental conditions B-cells and T-cells must share the same I region of the H-2 complex. Since hapten and carrier must be on the same molecule, the reaction of T_H with carrier and B-cell with hapten brings the helper and effector cells into close proximity. If they have I-region products which are identical, this allows the helper cell to signal the B-cell to become a functional effector cell.

Most immunologists agree that immunoglobulin (Ig) on the B-cell acts as antigen receptor, the argument being that the cell synthesizes the same antibody specificity that it uses to recognize and react with antigen at the cell surface. The B-cell has readily identifiable immunoglobulin on its surface, but the T-cell has little if any identifiable immunoglobulin on its surface. This poses the question of what kind of specific receptor molecule the T-cell uses to react with antigen. It has been postulated that some products of H-2 may be used as receptors by the T-cell. If this turns out to be true, it will provide a central role for the major histocompatibility complex because recent data suggests that the T-cell recognizes antigen if it is complexed to H-2 antigens, and then it is seen as altered self.

The key point of Section II is that helper and effector cells recognize and react with different antigenic determinants through specific cell surface receptors.

7

EFFECTOR AND HELPER CELLS IN ANTIBODY FORMATION: HAPTENS AND CARRIERS

OVERVIEW

In the preceding section we saw that cooperation between lymphocyte populations occurs in both antibody and cell-mediated responses. In this chapter and the next we will examine the role of antigen in these interactions. For antibody responses the notion will be developed that the thymus-derived cell and the bone marrow-derived cell each reacts with different antigenic determinants on the antigen molecule. These determinants are called haptens and carriers. We will show that T-cells react with carrier determinants and B-cells react with hapten determinants. Since T-cells are helper cells and B-cells are effector cells in antibody formation, this means that antibody is produced against the haptenic determinants and the carrier determinants are the helper determinants. This also means that an antigen molecule must be thought of as having two antigenic sites, the carrier sites which T-cells react with and the hapten sites which B-cells react with.

HAPTENS AND CARRIERS DEFINED

The key to understanding helper and effector cell interaction in antibody formation is the understanding of *haptens* and *carriers*. Historically the use of haptens was most fully exploited by Karl

Landsteiner (1868 to 1943). In his classic work *The Specificity of Serological Reactions* published in 1936 (and referred to in Chapter 1 where the topic of haptens and carriers was introduced), Landsteiner showed that antibody formation against a simple azo compound could be induced by conjugating the compound onto an immunogenic molecule such as serum protein. Although the simple azo molecule would not elicit antibody formation when injected alone, the azo-protein conjugate elicited the production of anti-azo antibodies as well as anti-protein antibodies when injected into animals. The notion that the small nonimmunogenic molecule was using the large immunogenic protein molecule as a CARRIER was thus developed. The molecule which derived immunogenicity by being conjugated to the carrier was termed the HAPTEN. Hapten-carrier conjugates are widely used today in determining the function of the various cells in the immune response.

In Figure 1 it is seen that injection of carrier alone yields anti-carrier antibody, but injection of hapten alone does not yield anti-hapten antibody. However, when the hapten is conjugated to the carrier, injection of the hapten-carrier complex yields both anti-hapten *and* anti-carrier antibodies. Conjugation of the hapten onto another carrier yields anti-hapten antibodies and anti-carrier antibody against the other carrier.

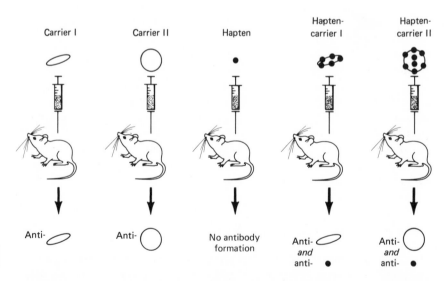

1

Antibody responses to carrier or hapten alone and carrier and hapten conjugates.

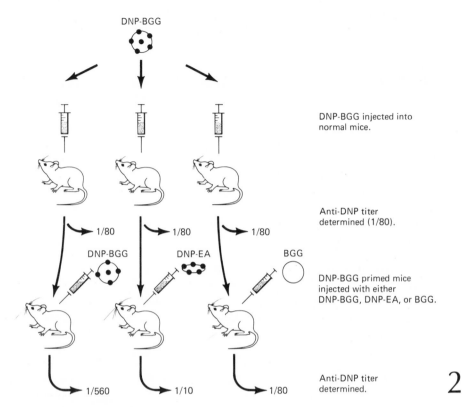

The carrier effect. [**After Ovary and Benaceraff (1963).** *Proc. Soc. Exp. Biol. Med.* **114, 72.**]

2

THE CARRIER EFFECT

The carrier portion of the immunogenic molecule plays more than a mere transport role as was originally thought. An example of what later came to be called the *carrier effect* is seen in the experiment in Figure 2. Dinitrophenyl (DNP) is a hapten which, when injected alone, does not result in antibody formation. Bovine gamma globulin (BGG) is a carrier which, when injected alone, results in anti-BGG antibody production. In these experiments rabbits were immunized with DNP conjugated to BGG. After suitable intervals the serum of the animals was assayed for anti-DNP antibody. The rabbits were then reinjected with either DNP-BGG (the homologous hapten-carrier protein), DNP-egg albumin (DNP-EA) (the same hapten on a heterologous carrier protein), or BGG (the carrier without the hapten). In the experiment shown, only the rabbits which received a second injection of DNP-BGG made a good secondary response to DNP. Thus even though all the animals had received a first injection of DNP (were primed to DNP), they made a secondary response to the second confrontation of DNP only when it was on the *same* carrier as the initial injection. This experiment shows that even though an animal is injected with the same hapten for both the primary and secondary responses, it will make a secondary or augmented response to the second injection of hapten only when the hapten is on the same carrier for both injections. This is called the carrier effect.

The explanation of the cellular basis of the carrier effect led to one of the central discoveries of modern immunobiology, that B-cells and T-cells react with different antigenic determinants on a molecule.

Adoptive Transfer of the Carrier Effect

For experimental analysis of the cell populations involved in the carrier effect Mitchison and his co-workers in London have used adoptive cell transfer experiments similar to those used in the reconstitution experiments described in Chapter 3. In these adoptive transfer experiments mice are lethally irradiated and injected with spleen cells from syngeneic mice. The donor mice have usually been primed to a hapten-carrier complex which we will call hapten-carrier-I (HC-I), and the repopulated mice are then challenged with HC-I or the hapten conjugated to a different carrier, which we will call hapten-carrier-II (HC-II). (In this case the second carrier is designated C-II.) A variety of experimental manipulations can be made on the spleen cells before transfer. By use of this experimental design the carrier effect can be transferred adoptively as seen diagrammatically in Figure 3.

Overcoming the Carrier Effect

We saw in the experiment in Figure 3 that the carrier effect could be transferred adoptively with spleen cells. The carrier effect can be overcome, i.e., a secondary response to HC-II can be obtained, if the recipient mice in the adoptive transfer are repopulated with hapten-carrier (HC-I) primed spleen cells *plus* cells from mice *primed to the heterologous carrier alone* (C-II). This is diagrammed in Figure 4.

Part A of this experiment is a repeat of the adoptive transfer of the carrier effect. In part B there are two groups of donors, one primed to HC-I and one primed only to the heterologous carrier, C-II. The irradiated recipients receive primed cells from each set of donors and are then challenged with hapten conjugated with the heterologous carrier (HC-II). The amount of anti-hapten antibody produced by these recipients is comparable with that in the mice in Figure 2

Mice injected with
nothing, HC-I or HC-II.

Spleen cells transferred
to irradiated recipients.
Challenged with HC-I.

Anti-
hapten   +   ++++   +
response

The transferred cells
show the carrier effect.

3

Adoptive transfer of the carrier effect.

which received homologous hapten-carrier injections. The C-II primed spleens could not be contributing the extra anti-hapten antibody because they were not primed to the hapten, but it is clear that they were necessary for the anti-hapten producing cells to be able to make their response.

This experiment shows some form of cooperation between the hapten-primed and the carrier-primed populations. It appears that when one set of cells is primed to hapten (HC-I) and one to carrier (C-II), they somehow interact to produce a secondary response to the hapten conjugated to the heterologous carrier. In other words, the carrier effect is overcome with carrier priming. The question becomes which cells react with hapten and which with carrier?

HAPTEN-REACTIVE AND CARRIER-REACTIVE LYMPHOCYTES

Anti-θ Treatment of Primed Cells

One of the landmark experiments in recent years was carried out in 1970 by Martin Raff in London. This experiment characterized the

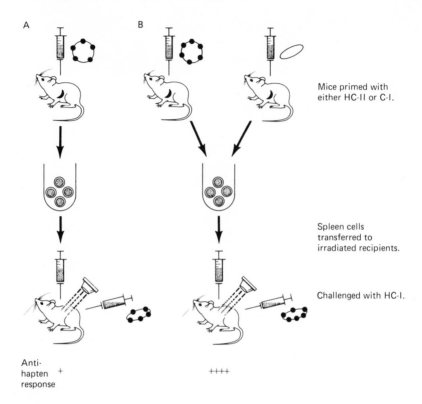

A

B

Mice primed with
either HC-II or C-I.

Spleen cells
transferred to
irradiated recipients.

Challenged with HC-I.

Anti-
hapten   +   ++++
response

4

Carrier priming overcomes the carrier effect in an adoptive transfer experiment.

interacting cells in the hapten-carrier response and paved the way for much of our understanding of B-cell and T-cell cooperation. The plan of the experiment is elegantly simple. It is essentially the carrier-priming experiment in Figure 4 with the additional step of treating the primed cells with either anti-θ or normal serum before transferring them to irradiated recipients. Treatment with anti-θ antiserum and complement will lyse T-cells so that it can be determined if the T-cells have responded to hapten or carrier.

The experiment and results are seen in Figure 5. In part A, one group of mice are primed with HC-I and another with C-II. After a suitable interval (approximately 1 week) the adoptive transfer is carried out. However, before transfer the carrier-primed cells are treated with anti-θ antiserum plus complement, and the hapten-primed spleen cells are treated with normal serum and complement. This means that all T-cells in the carrier-primed suspension are lysed, but the T-cells in the hapten-primed group are unaffected. The two populations are mixed and injected into irradiated hosts which are then challenged with hapten conjugated to carrier II (HC-II). Treating the carrier-primed population with anti-θ results in a poor anti-hapten response, which shows that anti-θ treatment abolished the ability to overcome the carrier effect. This means that the T-cells have reacted with the carrier.

In contrast, in part B, the hapten-primed spleen cells are treated with anti-θ antiserum plus complement, and the carrier-primed cells

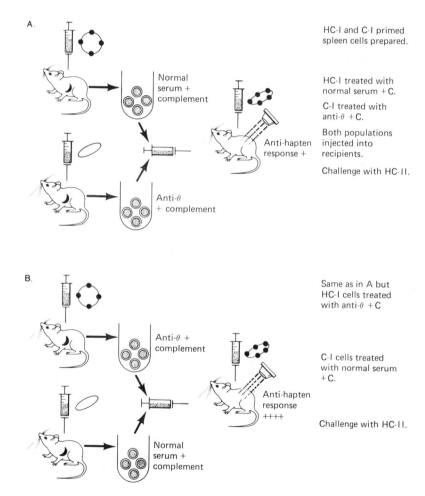

Experiment showing that carrier-primed cells are T-cells. [After Raff (1970). *Nature*, 226, 1257.]

5

with normal serum. In this case the carrier effect was overcome, showing that killing T-cells has no effect on the hapten-primed population. We know that antibody-producing cells are B-cells and that antibody is being produced against the hapten. Therefore this experiment dramatically shows that helper T-cells respond to carrier.

NATURE OF ANTIGENS

Carrier and Hapten Determinants on Antigens

Since most antigens are thymus-dependent, that is, require T-cell help for the appropriate stimulation of B-cells to produce antibody, this means that most antigens must contain both hapten and carrier determinants. Up to now we have used the term *antigen* as if it were a homogeneous substance. In fact, most common antigens, both soluble and particulate, have many *antigenic determinants*. The whole molecule can be called the *immunogen* to distinguish it from the separate determinants. In common use, however, immunologists refer to the whole molecule as antigen and call the separate antigenic moieties DETERMINANTS. Another term for antigenic determinants which is occasionally used is EPITOPE. One occasionally sees reference to epitope density, the number of identical antigenic determinants on an immunogen molecule.

While the question has not been answered, we will make the assumption that in one case a determinant can act as a hapten and in another case act as a carrier. Visualize a complex molecule with at least two antigenic determinants. If a T-cell reacts with determinant P and a B-cell reacts with determinant Q, this means that we will get anti-Q antibody. Q will be acting as a hapten, and since the helper T-cell reacted with P, that determinant must be acting as carrier (Figure 6). However, if a B-cell reacts with P and a T-cell with Q, then we will get anti-P. This makes the assumption that T-cells and B-cells have some overlapping repertoire of surface receptors for hapten and carrier. The nature of the receptors for the antigen on B-cells and T-cells will be covered in Chapter 10.

Thymus-Independent Antigens

Most antigens require T-cell help. Some, however, can induce antibody formation in the absence of T-cells. These are called *thymus-independent antigens*. There are several theories about the nature of thymus independency, but a thorough understanding of their subtleties requires a knowledge of possible modes of B-cell and

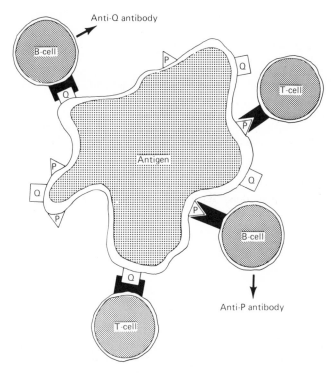

6

Hapten and carrier determinants on the same molecule.

T-cell interaction (which will be covered in Chapter 9). At this point we can explain one of the theories for thymus independency. Most, if not all, antigens which act in the absence of helper T-cells are composed of *repeating subunits* of the same antigenic determinant. The most commonly used thymus-independent antigens are polymerized flagellin (a protein of repeating subunits) or various polysaccharides (which are repeating units of sugars). The proponents of the theory which explains thymus-independency on the basis of repeating subunits argue that the signal to the B-cell which the T-cell gives in thymus-dependent responses involves the spatial rearrangement of receptors on the B-cell surface. In cases where all the antigenic determinants are identical and in an ordered array on the antigen, this brings the B-cell receptors into the proper alignment for triggering by antigen. In this manner helper and carrier determinants are identical molecules and assume unique function because of spatial arrangement.

SUMMARY

1. Historically haptens have been defined as small molecules which do not by themselves induce the formation of antibody but do when conjugated to a large immunogenic molecule called a carrier. Haptens can react with the anti-hapten antibody elicited by a hapten-carrier conjugate.

2. The carrier effect is the requirement for the hapten to be conjugated to the same carrier in both a primary and secondary injection. Conjugating the hapten to another carrier for the secondary response does not lead to a secondary anti-hapten response. The carrier effect can be adoptively transferred.

3. Priming with the other carrier overcomes the carrier effect.

4. When carrier-primed cells are treated with anti-θ and complement before adoptive transfer along with cells primed to hapten on heterologous carrier, the carrier effect is not overcome. This shows that T-cells are primed to carrier.

5. Antigens can be thought of as having two determinants. Haptenic determinants react with B-cells; carrier determinants react with T-cells.

READINGS

Mitchison, N. A. (1971). The carrier effect in the secondary response to hapten-protein conjugates. I. Measurement of the effect with transferred cells and objections to the local environment hypothesis, *Eur. J. Immunol.* **1,** 10.

———— (1971). The carrier effect in the secondary response to hapten-protein conjugates. II. Cellular cooperation, *Eur. J. Immunol.* **1,** 18. (Analysis of the carrier effect.)

————, Rajewsky, K., and Taylor, R. B. (1970). In J. Sterzl and I. Riha (ed.), *Developmental Aspects of Antibody Formation and Structure,* Prague, Academia Publishing House of Czechoslovak Academy of Sciences, 547. (An insightful analysis of the significance of the carrier effect in cell cooperation.)

Raff, M. C. (1970). Role of thymus-derived lymphocytes in the secondary humoral immune response in mice, *Nature,* **226,** 1257. (The paper which showed that T-cells react with carrier.)

8

EFFECTOR AND HELPER CELLS IN CELL-MEDIATED RESPONSES: LD AND SD ANTIGENS

OVERVIEW

In the last chapter we saw that in antibody formation the antigen molecules contained two types of antigenic determinants, carrier determinants with which helper cells react and hapten determinants with which effector cells react. A similar dichotomy of antigen function is also found in cell-mediated responses. The antigens used in cell-mediated responses are located on cell surfaces, and of these the antigens of H-2 complex are the most important. Antigens coded for the K and D regions of H-2 act as effector determinants in cytotoxic reactions, and antigens coded in the I region of H-2 act as helper determinants and stimulate mixed lymphocyte reactions. The mixed lymphocyte reaction responding cells and the helper cells for the cytotoxic effector cells both respond to one set of surface antigens, but it is not known if the MLR reactive cell is the helper cell. As noted in Chapter 6, the helper determinants are called LD or lymphocyte defined, and the effector determinants are called SD or serologically defined.

SUBPOPULATIONS OF T-CELLS

Helper and Effector T-Cells

We saw in Chapter 4 that there is T-cell:T-cell cooperation in the CML reaction. This was elegantly shown through the use of anti-Ly antiserum. In those experiments, it will be recalled, neither the Ly 1 nor the Ly 2, 3 T-cells alone were able to generate large numbers of CML effector cells. Combining the Ly 1 and the Ly 2, 3 populations, however, restored CML activity to levels comparible with those of the untreated cells. This experiment showed that there are helper and effector cells which are T-cells, but it did not determine which cell was the effector cell and which cell was the helper cell.

To determine which of these interacting T-cells is the helper and which is the CML reaction effector cell, the following experiment was performed (Figure 1). CML effector cells were prepared by culturing C57BL/6 lymph node T-cells with irradiated BALB/c cells as antigen. The C57BL/6 cells which are H-2^b react to the alloantigens on the BALB/c cells which are H-2^d, and the cytotoxic cells which are generated are assayed by ^{51}Cr release from BALB/c target cells. After the cytotoxic (or killer) cells have been generated but before the labeled target cells are added, the cells are treated with either anti-Ly 1 or anti-Ly 2, 3 antiserum and complement. In this manner, the Ly 1 cells are removed leaving Ly 2, 3 cells, or the Ly 2, 3 cells are removed leaving the Ly 1 cells. If either the Ly 1 or the Ly 2, 3 cells are the effector population, there should be a dramatic reduction in ^{51}Cr release after treatment with the appropriate antibody and complement.

The results of the experiment show that a reduction occurs after treatment with anti-Ly 2 or anti-Ly 3 but not after treatment with anti-Ly 1. Since the effector cells had already been generated before treatment with the antibody, this experiment shows that the *effector cell* in CML has Ly 2 and Ly 3 on its surface. Since we know that cells with Ly 1 act synergistically with the Ly 2, 3 cells, it follows that the *helper cell* in CML is an Ly 1 cell.

Helper Cell in CML and MLR Reactive Cell Compared

The results of the experiment in Figure 1 argue that Ly 1 positive cells are the helper cells in CML reactions. The following experiment shows that Ly 1 cells are cells which respond in MLR. It will be recalled from Chapter 4 that the MLR measures the amount of proliferation which a cell population has undergone in response to antigen. The experiments which tested the effect of anti-Ly antisera on MLR are diagrammed in Figure 2. In this experiment strain combinations were chosen in which K and D regions of H-2 were identical in both the responding population and the cells used as antigen, but the strains differed in the antigens of the I region. The responding cell population was treated with either anti-Ly 1, anti-Ly 2, or anti-Ly 3 *prior* to being mixed with the stimulator cells. In this way the Ly profile of the cells which initiate the MLR can be

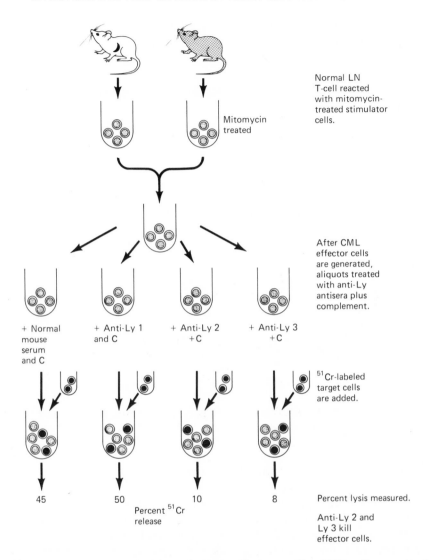

Normal LN T-cell reacted with mitomycin-treated stimulator cells.

Mitomycin treated

After CML effector cells are generated, aliquots treated with anti-Ly antisera plus complement.

+ Normal mouse serum and C

+ Anti-Ly 1 and C

+ Anti-Ly 2 +C

+ Anti-Ly 3 +C

^{51}Cr-labeled target cells are added.

45

50

10

8

Percent ^{51}Cr release

Percent lysis measured.

Anti-Ly 2 and Ly 3 kill effector cells.

1

Determining the Ly profile of CML effector cells. [After Cantor and Boyse (1975). *J. Exp. Med.* **141, 1376.]**

determined. After several days in culture tritiated thymidine was added, and the amount of label incorporated into DNA was determined. It can be seen in Figure 2 that treatment with anti-Ly 1 abolished the generation of MLR. Pretreatment with either anti-Ly 2 or Ly 3 had no effect. This shows that the cells which carry out an

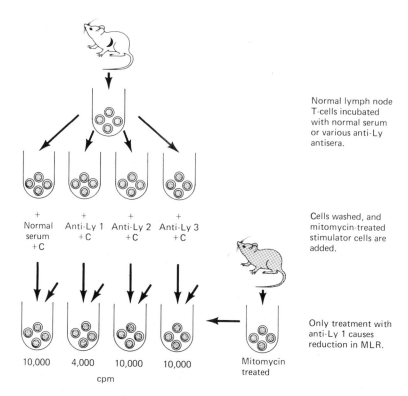

Normal lymph node T-cells incubated with normal serum or various anti-Ly antisera.

Cells washed, and mitomycin-treated stimulator cells are added.

Only treatment with anti-Ly 1 causes reduction in MLR.

2

Determining the Ly profile of MLR precursor cells. [After Cantor and Boyse (1975). *J. Exp. Med.* **141, 1376.]**

MLR to antigenic determinants of the I region have Ly 1 on their surfaces.

From the experiments in Figures 1 and 2 we see that Ly 2, 3 T-cells are effector cells in CML and the Ly 1 T-cells serve as helper cells. We also see that Ly 1 cells are MLR reactive cells. It is tempting to connect these two pieces of data and say that the MLR cell is the helper cell, but we cannot do this. Experiments must be carried out showing other similarities or differences between them.

Effector Cells in DTH

The experiments with CML showing effector cells bearing Ly 2, 3 and helper cells having Ly 1 on their surfaces immediately caused a sense of euphoria because they suggested that a pattern of helper- and effector-cell function was emerging. It was already known that the helper cell in antibody formation is Ly 1, and so it appeared that the general rule would be Ly 1 for helper cells and Ly 2, 3 for effector cells. The euphoria lasted only a few months because it was shown that the effector cell in *delayed-type hypersensitivity* is Ly 1.

It will be recalled from Chapter 4 that delayed-type hypersensitivity (DTH) is a reaction which is caused by T-cells in response to antigen. It is measured by injecting antigen into the skin of a primed animal and measuring the amount of swelling at the site 48 hr later. This reaction can be demonstrated in the mouse by using an adoptive transfer system in which mice are primed to an antigen and the T-cells injected into irradiated recipients. The recipients are then challenged with antigen, and the amount of swelling at the site of injection is measured. If the transferred cells are treated with either anti-Ly 1, Ly 2, 3, or normal serum before transfer, the Ly phenotype of the effector cell in DTH can be determined. By means of such an experiment, it was found that the DTH effector cell is Ly 1. This shows that there is no general rule of effector cells bearing Ly 2, 3 and helper cells bearing Ly 1.

Preferential MLR or CML Responses

The experiments described above showed that the helper cells in CML were Ly 1 and suggested that these cells were the cells which react in MLR. A long series of experiments by Fritz Bach and his co-workers in Madison, Wisconsin, have shown that there are separate subpopulations of T-cells which react with different antigens of the H-2 complex. The general plan of these experiments has been to test the ability to stimulate MLR of cells from strains of mice with known differences in the H-2 complex. For example, by choosing the proper congenic recombinants, it is possible to test the contribution to the MLR of an antigen difference in only the D region of H-2. To do this, one could choose as responder a strain which is, for example, bbbbbb. The stimulator cell (which is treated with mitomycin C) could then be bbbbbk. In this case the only difference is in the D region of the H-2 complex. Similar combinations can be set up for the K region and for the I region. The results of MLR stimulation studies are usually expressed as a stimulation index (SI) which is calculated as follows:

$$\frac{\text{cpm of experimental}}{\text{cpm of control}}$$

If the experimental incorporation is the same as the control, the SI is 1.0. If the experimental is six times the control, the SI is 6.0, etc.

When a large number of combinations were examined, a pattern emerged which is summarized in Table 1. This shows that the

TABLE 1.   EFFECT OF VARYING REGIONS OF H-2
COMPLEX ON GENERATION OF MLR.

Difference between responder and stimulator cells	Stimulation index
K	1.5
I	6.0
S	2.0
D	2.8

After Bach *et al.* (1972). *J. Exp. Med.* **136**, 1430.

greatest stimulation of the MLR is to differences at the I region of
H-2.

Similar kinds of experiments were also carried out in the CML
reaction, the idea being to vary only one region of H-2 and examine
the effect on CML. These results showed that differences at the I
region gave little or no CML but differences at the K and D regions
gave good stimulation. In all cases, however, differences at both K or
D *and* I gave the best results. These findings are summarized in
Table 2.

The "Three-Cell" Experiment

All the above data points to the fact that the helper determinants
are coded in the I region and appear on the T-cells which are active in
MLR. The effector determinants are coded in the K and D regions and
appear on T-cells which are active in CML. A good experiment to test

TABLE 2.   EFFECTS OF VARYING REGIONS
OF H-2 COMPLEX ON CML.

Difference between stimulator and responder cells	CML
K	Good
I	Poor
S	Poor
D	Good
K or D plus I	Very good

this notion is to add to a responder cell population one set of stimulator cells which differ only at K or D and another set of stimulator cells which differ only at I. The responder cell should give a good MLR to one, a fair CML to the other, and augmented CML and good MLR to the mixture of the two. This kind of experiment is called a "three-cell experiment." In the three-cell experiment shown in Figure 3 A is the responder cell and B and C are the mitomycin-C treated stimulator cells. A and B differ only at the I region, and the combination gives a good MLR but no CML. A and C differ at K and D, and this shows a moderate CML but a poor MLR. The mixture of the A plus B plus C gives good MLR and very good CML.

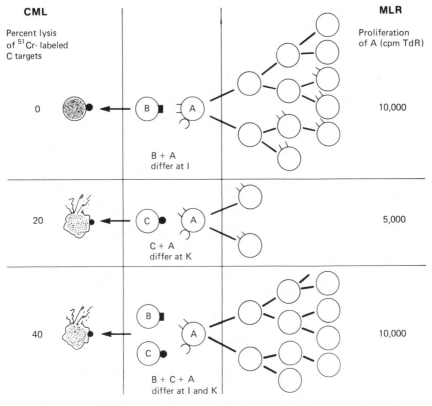

A three-cell experiment showing collaboration between cells with antigen B and antigen C in the generation of CML and MLR. [After Schendel and Bach, from Bach _et al._ (1976). _Nature_, 259, 273.]

3

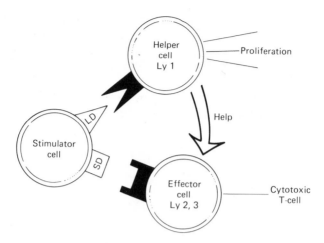

A model of effector and helper cell stimulation by LD and SD antigens.
[After Bach et al. (1976). Nature, 259, 274.]

4

LD AND SD ANTIGENS

The results of the kind of MLR and CML experiment in Figure 3
show that there is preferential stimulation of different T-cells by
antigens coded for in different regions of the H-2 complex. As noted
above, these antigens have been termed SD or serologically defined,
for the K- and D-region antigens and LD or lymphocyte defined, for
the I-region antigens. Some of the LD antigens are probably Ia
antigens. In the generation of cytotoxic cells which may be reactive to
tumors or grafts, both cells are needed for an optimum response. A
diagrammatic scheme is shown in Figure 4.

The analogy between helper and effector cells in cell-mediated
responses and helper and effector cells in antibody formation is
striking. In both cases two kinds of lymphocytes interact with two
kinds of determinants on the antigen, the result being a more efficient generation of effector cells.

SUMMARY

1. There are helper and effector populations in cell-mediated responses. The
   effector cell in CML is an Ly 2, 3 T-cell, and the helper cell is an Ly 1 cell.
   The effector cell in the delayed-type hypersensitivity responses is an Ly 1
   cell.
2. The cell which carries out MLR is an Ly 1 cell.

3. CML effector cells respond preferentially to K and D antigens on stimulating cells while MLR cells respond preferentially to I-region antigens.
4. The K and D antigens are called SD (serologically defined), and the I antigens are called LD (lymphocyte defined).
5. The dichotomy of response to antigen by effector and helper cells in cell-mediated responses is thus seen to be analogous to those in antibody formation.

READINGS

Cantor, H., and Boyse, E. A. (1976). Regulation of cellular and humoral immune responses by T-cell subclasses, in *Cold Spring Harbor Symposium on Quant. Biol.,* in press. (Review of subsets of T-cells based on Ly profiles.)

Bach, F. H., Bach, M. L., and Sondel, P. M. (1976). Differential function of major histocompatability complex antigens in T-lymphocyte activation, *Nature,* **259,** 273. (A clear exposition of cell cooperation and LD and SD antigens.)

Huber, B., Devinsky, O., Gershon, R. K., and Cantor, H. (1976). Cell-mediated immunity: Delayed-type hypersensitivity and cytotoxic responses are mediated by different T-cell subclasses, *J. Exp. Med.* **143,** 1534.

Vadas, M. *et. al.* (1976). Ly and Ia antigen phenotypes of T cells involved in delayed-type hypersensitivity and in suppression. *J. Exp. Med.* **144,** 10.

(Two papers which distinguish T-cell subclasses by surface antigens.)

9

MECHANISMS OF EFFECTOR- AND HELPER-CELL COOPERATION

OVERVIEW

So far we have developed the evidence that there are effector and helper cells in both antibody formation and cell-mediated responses. We know that in both situations there are helper determinants and effector determinants on the antigens. In this chapter, we will look at the bewildering array of data and models which try to explain how the helper and effector cells in antibody formation and cell-mediated responses interact with each other via haptens, carriers, and LD and SD determinants. There are two general classes of explanations. One argues for soluble factors and the other for cell contact as the means by which helper and effector cells interact. All the soluble factor models require the carrier portion of the antigen or the LD antigen to react with the specific receptor on the helper T-cell. As a result of this interaction in these models the helper T-cell produces a soluble substance which then reacts with the effector-cell precursor. The effector-cell precursor reacts with hapten or SD antigen and in the presence of the soluble factor from the T-cell becomes a functional effector cell. In cell contact models it is the carrier determinant which reacts with the helper T-cell and brings that cell in close association with the effector-cell precursor. The effector-cell precursor then reacts with the haptenic or SD determinant. This close association results in the generation of a functional effector cell. There is at the present no compelling reason to choose between these two types of models. This chapter will cover the evidence for both types of models of interaction.

NATURE OF HELP IN ANTIBODY FORMATION

Cell Contact vs. Soluble Factors

Because hapten and carrier must be linked to the same molecule (Chapter 7), the initial theory to explain the mechanism of T-cell help in antibody formation was by way of *antigen presentation* or *cell contact*. In this model (Figure 1), the carrier portion of the molecule is thought to react with antigen receptor on the T-cell. The hapten portion of the molecule is then "presented" to the antigen receptor on the B-cell. This causes the B-cell to proliferate and differentiate. The hapten and carrier parts of the molecule thus act as a bridge. Implicit in this model is the notion that the cells themselves come into very close proximity so that the complete "signal" to the B-cell could be due to either the orientation of the hapten portion of the antigen molecule or cell contact by the T-cell. In the current form of this theory, Ia antigens play a very important role.

On the other hand, another set of models hypothesizes B-cell: T-cell cooperation by means of *soluble factors* elaborated by the T-cell. In these models, the carrier portion of the antigen reacts with the T-cell, and as a result of this specific interaction, the T-cell elaborates a soluble substance which reacts with the B-cell. The B-cell must react with this T-cell factor and the hapten portion of the antigen for a complete signal to proliferate and differentiate. The most simple form of this model is shown in Figure 1. There are at least three major variants of soluble-factor models. All three share the common feature of postulating that a factor produced by the T-cell can substitute for the T-cell in carrying out helper function, but they differ in their idea of the nature of the factor. In one of the models, the soluble factor has no ability to bind specifically to antigen, in the others it does have antigen specificity. In one of the two models which postulate antigen specificity the factor is immunoglobulin, but in the other it is Ia.

At the present time, there is no *a priori* reason to accept any of the models completely, and we shall present them with as little bias as possible. In fact, parts of all of them may in the end turn out to be correct.

T-CELL HELP BY SOLUBLE FACTORS—ALLOGENEIC EFFECT MODEL

The first model we will discuss argues that T-cells carry out their helper function by elaborating a soluble factor. This model requires that antigen react with a T-cell via the antigen-specific receptor on

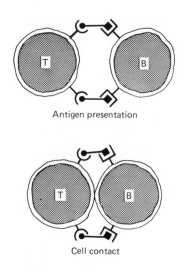

Antigen presentation

Cell contact

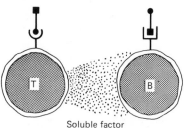

Soluble factor

Possible mechanisms of B-cell–T-cell cooperation.

the T-cell. This specific interaction causes the T-cell to elaborate a soluble factor. The key to the model is that once elaborated, the soluble factor can exert helper function to *any* B-cell as long as the B-cell reacts with antigen through its antigen-specific receptor molecules. The combination of soluble factor and antigen serves as the complete signal to the B-cell to proliferate and differentiate.

Allogeneic Effect

In the early middle ages of B:T interaction studies (*ca.* 1970) it was noted by Dutton and his co-workers that the ability of spleen cells from neonatally thymectomized mice to generate antibody responses could be restored *in vitro* by the addition of nonadherent (NA) cells from normal mice. This is not surprising since we know from Chapter 3 that NA cells contain T-cells. What was surprising was the fact that more antibody-forming cells were generated when allogeneic (cells from another strain of mice) T-cells were added than when syngeneic cells were used. This is seen in Figure 2.

A similar phenomenon was simultaneously and independently discovered by David Katz. (The number of times simultaneous observations occur points out again the futility of trying to assign precedence in an actively moving area. When an experiment's time has come, many bright people do it at the same time.) In this variant of the experiment (Figure 3) animals are primed with hapten-carrier I (HC-I). After a suitable interval one group of these primed animals is injected with HC-II, and, as expected, there is a weak secondary

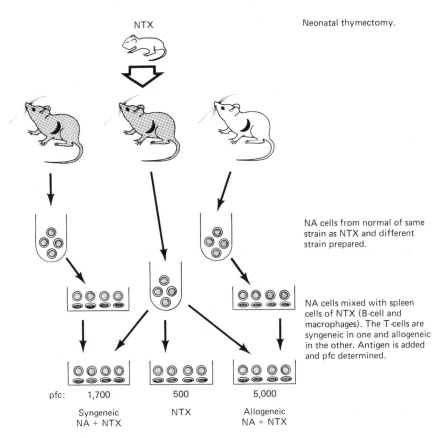

NTX

Neonatal thymectomy.

NA cells from normal of same strain as NTX and different strain prepared.

NA cells mixed with spleen cells of NTX (B-cell and macrophages). The T-cells are syngeneic in one and allogeneic in the other. Antigen is added and pfc determined.

pfc: 1,700   500   5,000

Syngeneic   NTX   Allogeneic
NA + NTX   NA + NTX

2

Allogeneic NA cells reconstitute neonatal thymectomized spleens better than syngeneic NA cells. [After Hirst and Dutton (1960). *Cell. Immunol.* 1, 190.]

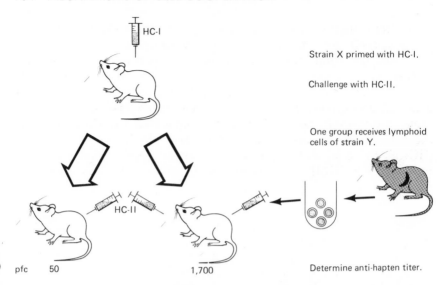

3

pfc 50 1,700

Strain X primed with HC-I.

Challenge with HC-II.

One group receives lymphoid cells of strain Y.

Determine anti-hapten titer.

The allogeneic effect. [After Katz *et al.* (1971). *J. Exp. Med.* 133, 169.]

anti-hapten response (i.e., the carrier effect). A second group of HC-I primed animals receives lymphoid cells from another strain (allogeneic cells) at the time they receive the challenge of HC-II. These animals produce a strong secondary anti-hapten response. In other words, the injection of the allogeneic cells allowed the carrier effect to be overcome. This ability of allogeneic cells to overcome the carrier effect is called the *allogeneic effect.*

Viable and immunocompetent cells are better able to carry out this overriding of the carrier effect than nonviable cells. Indeed, the carrier effect is best overcome under conditions in which a graft-versus-host reaction is occurring. We already know that the carrier portion of the antigen reacts with T-cells and that the carrier effect can be overcome with carrier priming. In the allogeneic effect, another T-cell reaction, the GVH reaction also overcomes the carrier effect. So we have two means by which T-cells overcome the carrier effect: one by specific expansion of carrier-reactive clones (carrier priming) and the other by nonspecific expansion of T-cell clones (the allogeneic effect).

Allogeneic-Effect Factor

It has been possible to substitute *supernates* of allogeneic cells for T-cells in carrying out allogeneic-effect experiments. In experiments of this type, F_1 spleen cells are incubated with parental spleen cells *in vitro.* The F_1 cells have antigens A and B on their surface, but the parental cells have only A *or* B antigen on their surfaces. The F_1 cells do not react against the parental cells because they do not see any foreign antigen. The parental cells which have antigen A see the B antigens as foreign and react to them. This form of reverse Oedipus complex is essentially the equivalent of a GVH reaction *in vitro.* Medium in which the cells were reacting is called the supernatant (supernate for short) of the reaction. If the supernate is collected and added to a culture of cells from which the T-cells have been removed by anti-θ treatment, the supernate substitutes for T-cells in generating helper function. These supernatant factors generated by allogeneic interactions are termed ALLOGENEIC-EFFECT FACTORS (AEF).

We thus have a situation in which the activation of T-cells by one set of antigens (alloantigens) allows the T-cells to elaborate a factor which can substitute for helper T-cells for a variety of thymus-dependent antigens. The elaboration of the factor by T-cells requires that a specific antigen react with the receptors on T-cells specific for that antigen. The factor which is produced, however, works for any other antigen. Because of this the factor is considered a *nonspecific factor.* Since the AEF is able to substitute for T-cells in giving helper function to B-cells, it is not unreasonable to assume that in nature the T-cell may carry out its helper role by the elaboration of this factor. An understanding of the chemical nature of the factor then becomes very important.

Nature of Allogeneic-Effect Factors

To determine if AEF is an immunoglobulin molecule or an H-2 product, the material was passed through an *immunoabsorbent column* containing either anti-Ig or anti-H-2. The rationale of the immunoabsorbent column is seen in Figure 4. Antibody molecules are covalently linked to an insoluble support such as Sepharose and poured into a column. If a solution containing an antigen which reacts with the antibody is passed down the column, the antigen will react with the antibody on the column. All materials in the solution which do not react with the antibody will pass through the column unimpeded. Thus, if a material is retained on the column, it has reacted with the antibody on the column, and material which passes through the column has not reacted with the antibody on the column.

When AEF was passed through an anti-Ig column, it was not retained, showing that it does not react with anti-Ig and therefore is not Ig in nature. However, when it was passed through an anti-H-2 column, it was retained, showing that it is made up of products of the H-2 complex. In these experiments, H-2^d T-cells from DBA/2 mice

4

The principle of an immunoabsorbent column.

were reacted with H-2$^{d/k}$ cells from (DBA/2 × C3H)F$_1$ mice. The H-2^d cells reacted to the H-2^k antigens on the F$_1$ cells so that the supernate contained AEF which was generated by the H-2^d cells.

To determine if AEF has active components which are products of either the K end (K and I regions) or the D end (S and D regions) of the H-2 complex, advantage was taken of antisera raised in congeneic mice (Chapter 6). In these mice, the background genes are identical but the H-2 genes differ. By immunizing appropriate strains, antibody is obtained which reacts with the products of various regions of the H-2 complex. For example, to make an antibody against the K end of the complex, one would choose mice which have the same D end but differ at the K end. An example of such an immunization is B10.A anti-B10.D2. Background genes are the same in these congenics, and so are the S and D regions of H-2. (B10.A is kkkddd, and B10.D2 is dddddd.) The resultant antiserum will therefore contain anti-K end antibodies. By similar reasoning, one can obtain anti-D end antibodies by immunizing B10.BR (kkkkkk) with B10.A (kkkddd).

A variety of antisera raised in such a manner have been tested on immunoabsorbent columns for their ability to remove AEF activity from allogeneic supernates. A summary of results is presented in Table 1. It can be seen in the table that only anti-I region antibodies are the specificities which remove activity from the supernate. The conclusion then is that the active component in AEF which substitutes for T-cells is a product of the I region of the H-2 complex.

Soluble Factor AEF Model

The model which is constructed from the above experiments argues that any antigen reacting with its proper specific T-cell results in the elaboration of the factor. For purposes of studying the phenomenon, it is easiest to produce the factor through an allogeneic effect because so many T-cells are responsive to tissue antigens. In nature, however, it is postulated that the factor elaborated in response to carrier determinants will be the same as those elaborated in response to allogeneic determinants. The model is diagrammed in Figure 5.

TABLE 1. REMOVAL OF AEF ACTIVITY BY ANTI-H-2 IMMUNOABSORBENT COLUMNS.

Specificity of antiserum on column	H-2 molecules which pass through the column	AEF activity of passed molecules
K, I, S, D	None	Removed
K, I	S, D	Removed
S, D	K, I	Present
K	I, S, D	Present
I	K, S, D	Removed

From Armerding, Sachs, and Katz, (1974). *J. Exp. Med.* **140**, 1717.

Antigen reacts with T-cells.

Soluble factor

T-cells elaborate soluble factor.

Factor reacts with B-cells.

Anti- ■   Anti- ▲

Any reacted B-cell which
reacts with its antigen responds.

5

Diagram of the AEF model of T-cell cooperation in which the T-cell carries out helper function by elaborating a nonspecific soluble factor.

IgT MODEL

In the allogeneic-effect model discussed above the soluble factor which is elaborated by the T-cell is not an immunoglobulin and has no antigen specificity. In the next soluble-factor model we will consider, the product of the T-cell is *antigen specific*. In this model, the factor will give T-cell help only for the antigen used to generate the factor.

In this model, of which Marc Feldmann and his co-workers are the primary proponents, the T-cell is thought to react with the carrier part of antigen via *specific immunoglobulin receptors* on the T-cell surface.[1] This T-cell associated immunoglobulin has been termed IgT. The antigen-IgT complex is postulated to be shed from the T-cells and absorbed onto the surface of a macrophage which then presents the hapten part of the antigen to the B-cell. The presentation of the

[1]The great controversy over the existence of Ig on the T-cell will be discussed in detail in Chapter 10.

IgT-antigen complex to the B-cell by the macrophage constitutes the complete signal to the B-cell to proliferate and differentiate.

Design of IgT Experiments

The experimental system used to arrive at the scheme described above is shown in Figure 6. In these experiments carrier-primed T-cells are incubated with normal or hapten-primed B-cells *in vitro*, but the *cell populations are separated from each other by cell-impermeable membranes*. In this manner, the two populations are in the same environment, but there is no cell contact. The carrier-

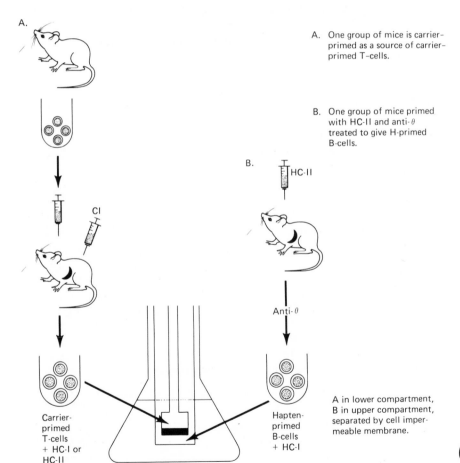

A. One group of mice is carrier-primed as a source of carrier-primed T-cells.

B. One group of mice primed with HC-II and anti-θ treated to give H-primed B-cells.

CI

B.

HC-II

Anti-θ

Carrier-primed T-cells + HC-I or HC-II

Hapten-primed B-cells + HC-I

A in lower compartment, B in upper compartment, separated by cell impermeable membrane.

6

Method used to test needs for cell contact between B-cells and T-cells. [After Feldmann and Basten (1972). *Nature, New Biol.* 237, 13.]

primed T-cells which are the source of helper T-cells are prepared by repopulating an irradiated mouse with thymus cells and then injecting the repopulated mouse with carrier. The sources of B-cells are spleen cells from mice which have been primed to a hapten. When these cells are treated with anti-θ and complement, only the B-cells remain. After a suitable interval the carrier-primed cells are cultured in one chamber of a Marbrook *in vitro* apparatus, and the hapten-primed, anti-θ treated cells are cultured in the other chamber with a cell-impermeable membrane between them. Antigen is present in both chambers. The fluids from the two chambers freely mix, but the cells do not contact each other because of the membrane. In this manner the need for cell contact or presence of a soluble factor can be determined.

By use of variants of this system, it was found that the B-cells were able to generate antibody under conditions in which the helper T-cells were physically separated from the B-cells. This shows that physical contact between B- and T-cells is not needed for the T-cell to carry out helper function, since the B-cells in the absence of T-cells across the membrane were not activated to produce antibody. The logical interpretation of these experiments is that a soluble factor has been elaborated by the T-cells after contact with antigen.

Antigen Specificity

The next question is how specific is this T-cell factor? Can T-cells primed to one antigen elaborate the factor in response to another antigen? To test this question, T-cells were primed to carrier I or carrier II and then incubated in the chambers across a membrane from B-cells primed to hapten and carrier I. The data in Table 2 shows that only the carrier to which the T-cells had been primed caused them to elaborate a factor which substitutes for helper T-cells when B-cells are challenged with HC-I. This argues that the factor has antigenic specificity.

TABLE 2.   SPECIFICITY OF SOLUBLE FACTOR IN Ig-T MODEL.

T-cells primed with	Antigen added to hapten-primed B-cells	Anti-hapten response
CI	HC-I	3,000
CII	HC-I	200

From Feldmann and Basten (1972). *J. Exp. Med.* **136**, 49.

Role of the Macrophage

In all the experiments described, there were *macrophages* in both compartments of the chambers. It was found that the system required the presence of macrophages. To determine the role of the macrophages, carrier-primed T-cells were incubated across a membrane from macrophages (rather than B-cells) as diagrammed in Figure 7.

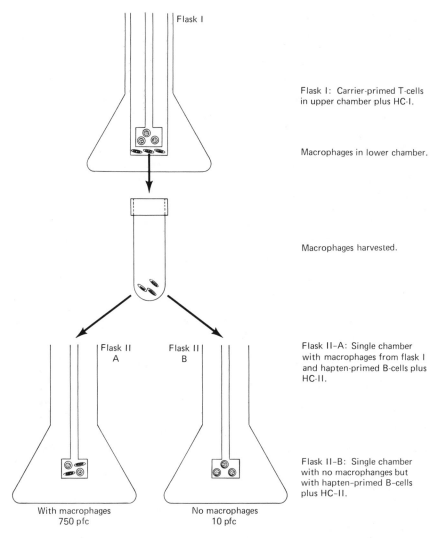

Flask I: Carrier-primed T-cells in upper chamber plus HC-I.

Macrophages in lower chamber.

Macrophages harvested.

Flask II-A: Single chamber with macrophages from flask I and hapten-primed B-cells plus HC-II.

Flask II-B: Single chamber with no macrophanges but with hapten-primed B-cells plus HC-II.

With macrophages
750 pfc

No macrophages
10 pfc

7

Two-chamber experiment to show the role of macrophages in the IgT-soluble factor system. [After Feldmann and Basten (1972).*J. Exp. Med.* 136, 737.]

In this experiment, the T-cell factors were allowed to diffuse across the membrane and react with the macrophages. The macrophages were then removed, washed, and cultured *in vitro* with B-cells. The data shows that the soluble factor which was elaborated by the T-cells is able to react with macrophages, and the macrophage-factor complex is able to substitute for T-cells. In the absence of macrophages the soluble factor has no effect on B-cells.

Nature of the Factor

The experiments above show that the soluble factor has antigen specificity and that it becomes associated with macrophages. But what is the chemical nature of the molecule which confers this specificity? Experiments in which anti-Ig was added to the culture showed that the specificity comes from *immunoglobulin*. This Ig is elaborated by the T-cell and so is called IgT. The evidence for this comes from experiments in which it was seen that the factor loses activity after being reacted with an anti-Ig antiserum. In these experiments, the factor was generated as in Figure 6 and then was reacted with anti-immunoglobulin. It was tested in the system in Figure 7 and had lost activity after anti-Ig treatment.

The model which was developed from this is shown in Figure 8. In this model antigen reacts with the T-cell which then sheds the antigen-IgT complex that becomes associated with the macrophage. The macrophage then presents the antigen to the B-cell.

Ia MODEL

A variant of the IgT soluble-factor model has been worked out by Munro and Taussig. In this model the factor from the T-cell is antigen specific but is not an immunoglobulin. Analysis shows, rather, that the factor is an H-2 product. The method used to arrive at this conclusion is diagrammed in Figure 9. Lethally irradiated mice are repopulated with thymus cells and then injected with antigen. The spleens of these mice serve as a source of primed T-cells. The primed T-cells are incubated *in vitro* for 6 to 8 hr with the same antigen used for priming. The T-cells are then removed, leaving a supernate. This supernate and normal bone marrow cells (the source of B-cells) are then injected into lethally irradiated recipients which are challenged with antigen. The ability of these bone marrow reconstituted mice to produce antibody-forming cells is then tested. In these experiments, TGAL (tyrosine-glutamic-alanine-lysine), a branched-chain synthetic antigen, was used (see Chapter 19). It can be seen in the figure that a soluble factor is elaborated by the primed thymus cells which reacts

T-cell reacts with carrier part of the antigen via immuno-globulin (IgT).

IgT-Ag complex is shed and reacts with macrophage.

Macrophage presents hapten part of the antigen to B-cell.

B-cell produces antibody.

Antibody production

8

Diagram of the IgT model of antigen-specific soluble T-cell product in B-cell–T-cell cooperation.

with B-cells so that the B-cells, when injected into the lethally irradiated hosts that have been treated with soluble factor, are able to respond to antigen by producing antibody. Thus, we have another case of a soluble factor being elaborated by the T-cell which substitutes for T-cell helper function.

Specificity of the Factor

To determine if this factor is specific, thymus cells from TGAL-primed mice were incubated *in vitro* with the specific antigen (TGAL). The supernate was then injected along with bone marrow cells plus TGAL into irradiated hosts as in Figure 9. The recipients were then challenged with TGAL (the specific antigen) or SRBC (a

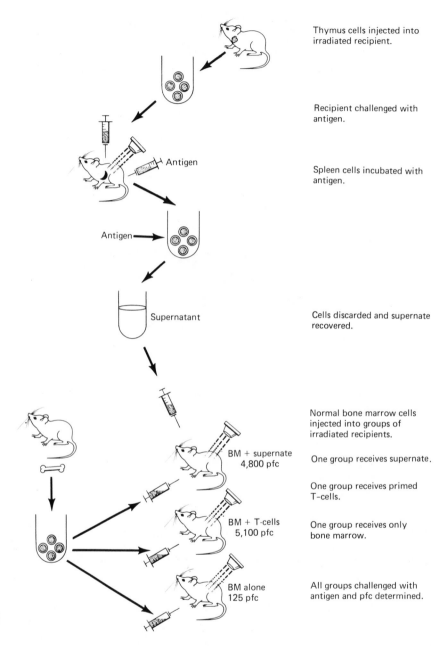

Thymus cells injected into
irradiated recipient.

Recipient challenged with
antigen.

Spleen cells incubated with
antigen.

Cells discarded and supernate
recovered.

Normal bone marrow cells
injected into groups of
irradiated recipients.

One group receives supernate.

One group receives primed
T–cells.

One group receives only
bone marrow.

All groups challenged with
antigen and pfc determined.

9

Generating and testing the T-cell factor in the Ia model system. [After Taussig (1974). *Nature*, 248, 234.]

nonspecific antigen). The results in Table 3 show that the factor possesses antigen specificity as judged by the fact that the mice which received TGAL made anti-TGAL responses but the recipients challenged with SRBC did not produce anti-SRBC antibody. This indicates that the factor is not able to act nonspecifically, making it similar to the IgT factor but different from AEF.

Nature of the Factor

We saw in the IgT model of specific soluble factors that the antigen-specific soluble factor was immunoglobulin. Since the factor in this system is also specific (Table 3), to determine if it also derives its specificity by being immunoglobulin, it was passed through an immunoabsorbent column containing either anti-mouse Ig or anti-H-2 as in the AEF studies described above. The material which passed through the column was then injected, along with bone marrow cells, into irradiated animals. In this way, if the active material in the supernate was Ig, it would be retarded by the anti-Ig column and the material that passes through the column would not have activity when injected into recipients along with bone marrow.

TABLE 3.   SPECIFICITY OF T-CELL SUPERNATE IN Ia MODEL OF B:T COOPERATION.

Irradiated recipients injected with	*Antigen*	*Anti-SRBC pfc*	*Anti-TGAL pfc*
B-cells	SRBC	130	—
B-cells + normal T-cells	SRBC	2,560	—
B-cells + TGAL primed T-cells	SRBC	116	—
B-cells + supernate produced by TGAL primed T-cells	SRBC	84	—
B-cells	TGAL	—	250
B-cells + supernate produced by TGAL primed T-cells	TGAL	—	3,970

After Taussig (1974). *Nature,* **248,** 234.

As seen in the data in Table 4, the anti-Ig column did not remove activity but the anti-H-2 column did. Thus, this material appears to differ from the IgT factor since it is not an immunoglobulin. However, it is similar to AEF because it contains H-2 molecules. In experiments carried out to localize the factor within the H-2 complex, it was possible to localize activity of the factor to the IA subregion of H-2.

A schematic representation of this model is seen in Figure 10.

SUMMARY OF SOLUBLE-FACTOR MODELS

Table 5 contains a summary of some of the pertinent points concerning the soluble T-cell factors we have been discussing. It is obvious that the models are still more like jigsaw puzzles with missing pieces than complete pictures. They have pieces in common, but they also have pieces which are different. At this point, we do not know which parts of the models are relevant to the way the immune system works *in vivo* under natural conditions and which parts are artifacts of the methods. There is the possibility that all three are correct because the immune system has evolved several ways of attaining a common end.

CELL CONTACT MODELS OF B:T COOPERATION

Experimental Design

As we stated earlier, hapten and carrier must be on the same molecule to elicit a secondary anti-hapten response. The first model to explain this fact and other hapten carrier phenomena was an antigen

TABLE 4.   IMMUNOABSORBENT COLUMN
REMOVAL OF ACTIVITY OF
SOLUBLE FACTOR IN Ia MODEL.

Antiserum on column	Factor removed
Ig	No
H-2	Yes
K, IA, IB	Yes
IC, S, D	No
K	No
IA, IB, IC, S	Yes
IB, IC, S, D	No

After Taussig *et al.* (1975). *J. Exp. Med.* **142,** 694.

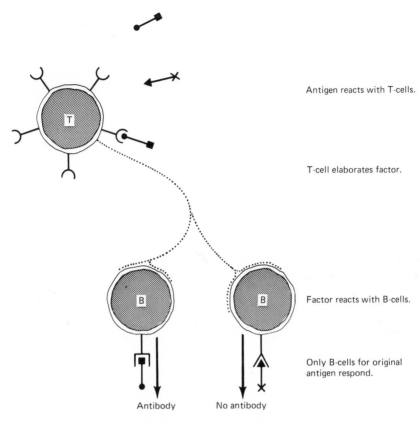

Antigen reacts with T-cells.

T-cell elaborates factor.

Factor reacts with B-cells.

Only B-cells for original antigen respond.

Antibody   No antibody

10

Schematic representation of soluble T-cell product with antigen specificity which is Ia in nature.

TABLE 5.   SUMMARY OF SOLUBLE-FACTOR MODELS BY T-CELL HELP IN ANTIBODY FORMATION.

	AEF	*IgT*	*Ia*
Produced by T-cells	Yes	Yes	Yes
Antigen specific	No	Yes	Yes
Chemical nature	H-2 (I)	Ig	H-2 (IA)
Binds to antigen	No	Yes	Yes

presentation or a cell contact model. According to this notion the carrier portion of the antigen molecule reacts with the T-cell which then presents the hapten portion to the B-cell. To do this, the T-cell comes into close proximity with the B-cell. With the experiments showing that T-cells could cooperate with B-cells across cell-impermeable membranes and that soluble supernatant factors could also substitute for T-cells, this notion fell upon hard times.

Recent experiments, however, have resurrected a sophisticated variant of this model. One of the unexpected results of the original marrow-thymus studies (Chapter 3) was that allogeneic bone marrow and thymus cells would not cooperate in irradiated hosts. In further analyzing this result, it is possible to test whether background or H-2 differences play a role in preventing cooperation by using congenic mice which have identical H-2 and different background genes or vice versa as the sources of the interacting cells. For example, if the B-cell donor is strain A and the T-cell donor B10.A, both have identical H-2 regions (kkkddd) but differ at all background genes. These cells are injected into irradiated (B10.A × A)F$_1$ mice to determine if they can cooperate in antibody formation. Their ability or failure to cooperate tells us if H-2 or background genes are important in the interaction. The basic design of these experiments which have been carried out by Katz and his collaborators is seen in Figure 11. In a typical experiment nonirradiated (B10.A × A)F$_1$ mice were recipients which were repopulated with carrier-primed cells from B10.A. They were then X-irradiated and given hapten-primed B-cells (anti-θ treated HC-II primed cells) and challenged with HC-I. This design is possible because helper T-cells can carry out help after irradiation if they have been exposed to antigen and allowed to proliferate before irradiation.

It can be seen in Figure 12 that when the cells were from the same strain (B10.A) there was good cooperation as expected. When the cells were from different strains (B10.A and A.By), there was very poor cooperation. The crucial groups here are groups III and IV. In group III the H-2 regions are identical but the backgrounds are different (B10.A and A) and there is good cooperation. In group IV, however, the backgrounds are identical (B10 and B10.A) with H-2 different and this results in poor cooperation. From this kind of experiment it was concluded that similarities in H-2 are required for B-cell:T-cell cooperation.

The experiment in Figure 12 shows that B- and T-cells can cooperate when background genes are different but H-2 genes are identical. Experiments of similar design but using other recombin-

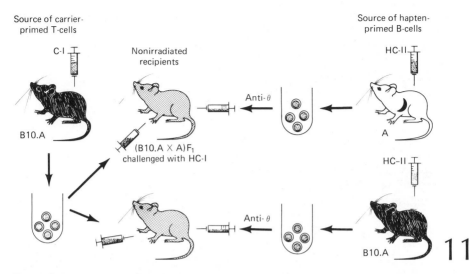

Experimental design for testing cooperation between same H-2 and different backgrounds. By choice of appropriate strain combinations, other genetic loci can be tested. [After Katz *et al.* (1973). *P.N.A.S.* 70, 2624.]

	B-cells	T-cells	Genetic difference	Anti-hapten antibody produced
I	B10.A kkkddd	B10.A kkkddd	H-2 same, background same	
II	B10.A kkkddd	A.By bbbbbb	H-2 different, background different	
III	B10.A kkkddd	A kkkddd	H-2 same, background different	
IV	B10.A kkkddd	B10 bbbbbb	H-2 different, background same	

B-cell–T-cell cooperation across identical and dissimilar H-2 backgrounds. [After Katz *et al.* (1973). *P.N.A.S.* 70, 2624.]

ants showed that the crucial differences in the H-2 complex are localized in the I region. The results of these experiments are summarized in Table 6.

Interpretation

An interpretation of these experiments has been advanced that the I-region genes code for products which are necessary in B-cell and T-cell cooperation. These genes are termed CELL INTERACTION (CI) genes. It is postulated that CI genes code for surface molecules which must be identical for the B- and T-cells to interact. Presumably the necessity for the identity is to facilitate cell-to-cell interaction. This could be physical contact or membrane interactions at very close distance.

Histoincompatible Cell Cooperation in Chimeras

It is possible, however, to get histoincompatible B-cell and T-cells to cooperate. One means of doing this is by producing tetraparental or allophenic mice. These mice are produced by fusing the eight-cell-stage embryo of two different mice and reimplanting the cells into a pseudopregnant mother. The mice that develop are CHIMERAS; i.e., the cells of both embryos are growing side by side in the same animal. It can be shown that any individual cell is derived from one set of parents and another cell is from the other set of parents. If one of the parents was H-2^b and the other was H-2^k, then the mouse would have H-2^b and H-2^k cells living adjacent to each other. In such animals histoincompatible B-cells and T-cells have been shown to interact and produce antibody.

TABLE 6.   DIFFERENCES WITHIN THE I REGION
AND B-CELL AND T-CELL
COOPERATION.

H-2 differences between B-cells and T-cells	Cooperation
K, S	Yes
K	Yes
S	Yes
I, S	No
K, I, S	No
I, S, D	No
D	Yes

After Katz *et al.* (1975). *J. Exp. Med.* **141**, 263.

Another means of producing chimeras is to repopulate an irradiated F_1 mouse with bone marrow of the parental strains. In the experiments described below (CBA × DBA/2)F_1 mice were repopulated with bone marrow from the parental strains CBA and DBA/2. These mice were shown 2 to 7 months later to have approximately equal numbers of CBA lymphocytes and DBA/2 lymphocytes. It is important to remember that this situation is different from that of an F_1 of CBA and DBA/2, where each of the lymphocytes would have *both* CBA and DBA/2 antigens. In chimeras the CBA and DBA/2 cells live side by side, and each cell has *either* CBA or DBA/2 antigens.

By using appropriate anti-H-2 and anti-θ antisera, it is possible to obtain CBA B-cells and DBA/2 T-cells (and vice versa) from the chimeras. When these cells were used in B-cell:T-cell cooperation experiments, it was found that they were able to cooperate as well as syngeneic cells. This means that histoincompatible B-cells and T-cells obtained from long-term chimeras were able to interact across a histocompatibility barrier.

This observation clearly raises questions about the need for I-region identity. What has changed in the cells obtained from the chimeras to make them function differently than the B-cells and T-cells which showed a need for I-region identity? There are several alternative explanations. A change could have occurred in the cells in the chimera during the several months of their side-by-side existence. For example, the cells perhaps could have become mutually tolerant of each other, i.e., lost the ability to respond to each other (see Chapter 20). In the short-term experiments where no cooperation for antibody was seen, there could have been a reaction of the interacting cells (an MLR, for example) which prevented them from cooperating for antibody formation. Similarly, suppressor cells could have been generated (Chapter 18).

Another explanation which is worth considering is the possibility that the cells in the chimera are at a different stage of differentiation. In the short term or acute experiments (Figure 11) the B-cells and T-cells were at a stage of differentiation which did not allow them to cooperate across I-region barriers. In the chimeras they could have differentiated to a point where they are able to carry out cooperation across the I region. This postulated change has been termed *adaptive differentiation*.

CURRENT STATUS

It is clear from the mass of data and the several models presented in this chapter that we can currently draw no hard and fast conclusion about the manner in which effector and helper cells cooperate. Helper cells may exert their influence on effector cells by one or many soluble factors and/or by cell contact. This is a field of intense research, and very likely the separate lines of evidence will begin to come together in a more comforting pattern before this text is in its second edition.

MECHANISM OF INTERACTION IN CML

With the realizations that a soluble factor can replace the helper cell in antibody reactions and that there is similarity between the helper-effector cell relationship in cell-mediated responses, many groups are now beginning to look at the nature of the interaction in CML. One recent report by Janet Plate shows that a soluble factor liberated by T-cells can substitute for helper cells. In these experi-

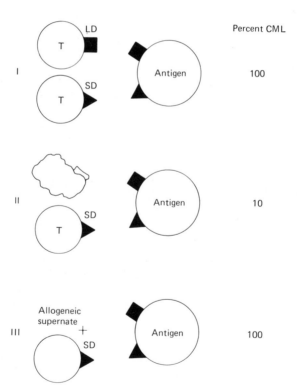

13

Soluble T-cell factor replaces helper cell in CML. [After Plate (1976). *Nature*, 260, 329.]

ments the helper cells were removed by treatment with an antiserum directed against them. In the CML reaction the helper cell was replaced by the supernate of a reaction of B10 cells with irradiated B10.D2 cells. This supernate replaced the need for helper T-cells in the CML (Figure 13).

It will be interesting to see if other factors are discovered in T-cell:T-cell cooperation and if they have as many apparently contradictory characteristics as those in T-cell:B-cell interactions.

SUMMARY

1. There are two broad classes of theories which explain the nature of the interaction between helper T-cells and effector B-cells. In one of these the T-cell elaborates a soluble factor which interacts with the B-cell, in the other cell contact is needed.

2. There are three soluble-factor models currently under consideration. *Allogeneic-effect factor (AEF) model:* In this model the carrier portion of the antigen is thought to react with T-cells specific for the carrier. These T-cells then elaborate a soluble factor, called allogeneic-effect factor. The reaction of the B-cell with hapten and AEF signals the B-cell to proliferate and differentiate into an antibody-forming cell. The soluble factor is not antigen specific and is a product of the I region of the H-2 complex.

   IgT model: According to this model the carrier portion of the antigen reacts with the specific T-cells through IgT, an antibody molecule at the T-cell surface. The antigen-IgT complex is shed from the T-cell surface and reacts with a macrophage, which then presents the hapten portion of the antigen to the B-cell. The soluble factor in this model is antigen specific and is an immunoglobulin.

   Ia model: This model holds that the carrier portion of the antigen molecule reacts with the specific T-cell, causing the T-cell to liberate a soluble factor which reacts with B-cells. The soluble factor in this model is antigen specific and is a product of the I region of the H-2 complex.

3. The cell contact model is based on the fact that in some experimental conditions T-cells and B-cells must be syngeneic in the I region of the H-2 complex. It is postulated that some I-region products act as cell interaction regulators during cell contact, which is brought about by the hapten and carrier portions of antigen bridging the two cells.

4. Helper function in T-cell: T-cell cooperation in CML reactions appears to be carried out by a soluble factor.

READINGS

REVIEWS

Katz, D. H., and Benacerraf, B. (1972). The regulatory influence of activated T-cells and B-cell responses to antigen, *Adv. Immunol.* **15,** 2.

―――― and ―――― (1974). The role of histocompatability gene products in cooperative cell interaction between T and B-lymphocytes, in *The Immune System: Genes, Receptors, Signals, Proc. 1974 I.C.N.–U.C.L.A. Symposium on Molecular Biology*, E. Sercarz, A. R. Williamson, and C. F. Fox (eds.), New York, Academic Press.

Feldmann, M. *et al.* (1974). Interactions between T and B-lymphocytes and accessory cells in antibody production, in Brent and Holborow (eds.), *Prog. Immunol. II*, **3**, 65.

Munro, A. J. and Taussig, M. J. (1975). Two genes in the major histocompatability complex control immune response, *Nature*, **256**, 103.

ARTICLES

Taussig, M. J. (1974). T cell factor which can replace T cells *in vivo, Nature*, **248**, 234.

Feldmann, M. (1972). Cell interactions in the immune response *in vitro*. II. Specific collaboration via complexes of antigen and thymus-derived cell immunoglobulin, *J. Exp. Med.* **136**, 737.

Armerding, D., Sachs, D. H., and Katz, D. H. (1974). Activation of T and B lymphocytes *in vitro*. III. Presence of Ia determinants on Allogeneic Effect Factor, *J. Exp. Med.* **140**, 1717.

Katz, D. H., Dorf, M. E., and Benacerraf, B. (1974). Cell interactions between histoincompatible T and B lymphocytes. VI. Cooperative responses between lymphocytes derived from mouse donor strains differing at genes in the S and D regions of the H-2 complex, *J. Exp. Med.* **140**, 290.

(These papers are representative of the major viewpoints on T- and B-cell cooperation.)

Plate, J. M. D. (1976). Soluble factors substitute for T-T cell collaboration in generation of T-killer lymphocytes, *Nature*, **260**, 329. (A soluble factor in T-T helper function.)

10

RECEPTORS AND SIGNALS

OVERVIEW

Effector and helper cells react with different parts of the antigen molecule and carry out different functions. Both of these cells react specifically with antigen through antigen-specific receptors in their membranes. It is rather generally agreed that immunoglobulin is the receptor for antigen on B-cells, but the nature of the T-cell receptor is in dispute. The reaction between receptor and antigen must in some way signal the cell to begin carrying out its function, but we know very little of the nature of the signal. Recent data has shown that the recognition of "altered self" may be important in initiating responses to antigen.

PRECURSORS OF ANTIBODY-FORMING CELLS

The basis of clonal selection is that there are small numbers of cells committed to react with a specific antigen. The reaction of antigen with these cells induces them to proliferate (Chapter 17), thus expanding the clone of reactive cells. Two of the essential elements of the theory obviously must be that there are a small number of committed cells and that these cells can react specifically with antigen. The proof that these cells do indeed exist is given in the experiments below. The cells which are committed to react with a certain antigen are called ANTIGEN-REACTIVE CELLS. These antigen-reactive cells can be either *precursors* of effector cells or helper cells.

Assay of Precursors

The number of precursors of antibody-forming cells or cells pre-committed to respond to an antigen is determined *in vivo* by a *focus-forming assay*. An *in vitro* method will be discussed in Chapter 12. The principle of the focus-forming assay is based on the assumption that a single precursor cell is the precursor to the large number of antibody-forming cells seen after antigenic stimulus. This is reasonable since antigenic stimulation induces proliferation. In the spleen, the daughter cells which are the result of this proliferation remain localized at one site for a period of time and form active areas of antibody-forming cells similar to spleen colonies of hematopoietic cells. The experiment to measure the number of precursors (Figure 1) is analogous to the stem cell assay. Mice are lethally irradiated and repopulated with small numbers of spleen cells and antigens. A portion of the antigen-reactive cells in the population of the injected cells will lodge in the spleen of the recipient and proliferate in response to antigen. The clusters of antibody-forming cells which results is visualized by slicing the spleen into chunks, placing the chunks on an agar-SRBC layer, and adding complement. If there are antibody-forming cells in a piece of spleen, they will liberate antibody to react with the SRBC which will then be lysed by the complement. By looking for an area of hemolysis around a chunk of spleen, one can determine if there are antibody-forming cells in the chunk.

Since the number of cells which were injected is known, by counting the number of foci (areas of hemolysis) per spleen it is possible to calculate the number of precursor cells for the antigen in a normal spleen. The value obtained for SRBC and several other common antigens is between 10^{-6} and 10^{-5}. In other words, for every 10^6 spleen cells there is 1 precursor cell reactive to SRBC. This kind of experiment lends support to the notion that there are small numbers of cells reactive to antigen and that the progeny of these cells are an expanded clone.

Number of Cells Carrying Out GVH Reactions

One of the original arguments for having reservations about the clonal selection theory as it was initially formulated by Burnet was that the number of cells able to carry out a GVH reaction was far in excess of the small numbers of preprogrammed cells for an antigen which the theory predicted. Simonsen, using chickens, showed that as few as 50 parental cells injected into F1 embryos were able to induce a GVH reaction. If so few cells are able to induce the reaction, then clearly one of the main assumptions of the clonal selection notion

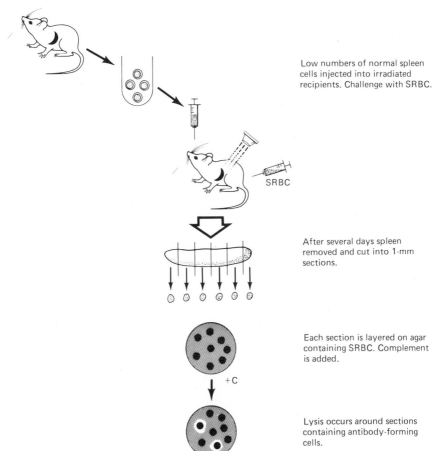

In vivo **focus-forming assay method of enumerating precursors of antibody for antibody-forming cells. [After Kennedy *et al.* (1965). *Proc. Soc. Exp. Biol. Med.* 120, 868.]**

Low numbers of normal spleen cells injected into irradiated recipients. Challenge with SRBC.

After several days spleen removed and cut into 1-mm sections.

Each section is layered on agar containing SRBC. Complement is added.

Lysis occurs around sections containing antibody-forming cells.

must be questioned. We have seen above that a small number of functional cells are reactive in antibody formation (and will see more about the number of developing clones in Chapter 12). But the numbers of cells in GVH reactions is an unexplained, often observed fact of life. At the end of this chapter very recent ideas of the nature of recognition and the need for recognizing altered self will be presented which take advantage of this fact.

Antigen Binding at the Cell Surface

The precursor of the antibody-forming cell responds to antigen. Presumably, this is done by specific antigen binding at the cell surface. An experiment which demonstrates that lymphocytes do in fact bind antigen at their cell surfaces is seen in Figure 2. In this experiment spleen cells from a normal mouse were incubated with antigen which had been radiolabeled with ^{125}I. The cells were allowed to react with the antigen for varying periods of time and were then washed and prepared for autoradiography. When they were examined in the microscope, the number of antigen-binding cells was found to be between 500 and 1,500 per 10^5 lymphocytes. This is a frequency of 10^{-2} (1 cell in 100), or anywhere from 100 to over 1,000 times greater than would be predicted from the number of *functional* antigen-reactive cells as determined in the focus-forming cell studies mentioned above.

The conclusion drawn from these experiments is that more cells bind antigen than specifically respond to it. This could be because only one kind of effector cell is being assayed in the functional assay and the direct binding assay also determines antigen binding by other effector cells and by helper cells as well. It is also possible that some of the cells binding antigen are binding it nonspecifically. It is therefore crucial to show that among the many cells which bind

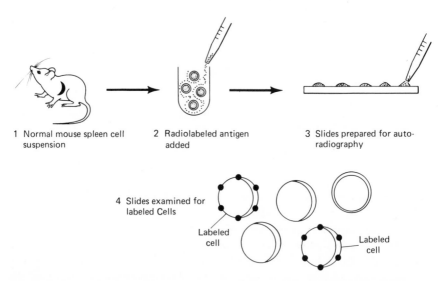

1 Normal mouse spleen cell
  suspension

2 Radiolabeled antigen
  added

3 Slides prepared for autoradiography

4 Slides examined for
  labeled Cells

Labeled
cell

Labeled
cell

2

Method for identifying antigen-binding cells. [After Ada (1970). Transplant. Rev. 5, 105.]

antigen there are some which bind it specifically (presumably via a surface receptor).

Specific Antigen Binding by Functional Cells

Since functional analysis predicts a frequency of 1 reactive cell per 10^5 or 10^6 cells and autoradiographic studies show 1 reactive cell in 10^2, it becomes important to have one assay which takes advantage of antigen-binding and functional analysis. This kind of assay was done by passing cells through columns coated with antigen and showing that specific reactive cells are retained by the column while other cells pass through. The experiment is shown in Figure 3. In this experiment insoluble beads were coated with antigen and then poured into a column. Normal spleen cells were then passed through the column of antigen-coated beads. If a cell has a surface receptor which reacts with the antigen on the column, the cell will be retarded in its passage through the column. If it does not react with the antigen, it will pass through the column unimpeded. The cells which passed through (i.e., those which have not reacted with antigen) were recovered and injected into irradiated mice which were challenged with the same antigen used on the column. If there are cells in the normal population able to specifically bind to antigen, then the cells which pass through the column should be devoid of cells able to react with antigen. This is exactly what happened in the experiment in Figure 3. The population which passed through the column of antigen was depleted of effector cells for the antigen on the column but had normal numbers of cells for a nonrelated antigen. This experiment shows that the functionally reactive lymphoid cells in the population can bind antigen specifically.

Antigen Binding by B- and T-Cells

Since functionally active cells bind antigen specifically, it is very important to know if both B-cells and T-cells are able to bind antigen. This question was answered with the following experiment. Since lymphocytes bind radiolabeled antigen, if the antigen that is used has been labeled with extremely high specific activity of radiolabel, the radiation damage to the cell after antigen binding should cause the cell to be specifically inactivated. This is called the ANTIGEN SUICIDE TECHNIQUE. In the experiment (Figure 4), thymus cells or B-cells (spleens from bone marrow repopulated, irradiated, thymectomized mice) were treated with antigen radiolabeled with high specific activity or with nonradioactive antigen. The principle of the experiment is that the great amount of radiation liberated at the cell surface by the bound labeled antigen will damage the lymphocytes which have

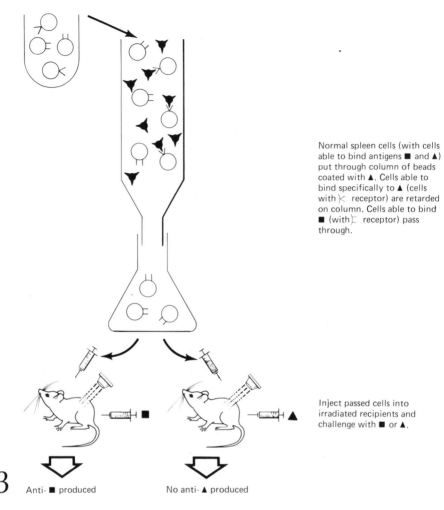

Normal spleen cells (with cells able to bind antigens ■ and ▲) put through column of beads coated with ▲. Cells able to bind specifically to ▲ (cells with ⊱ receptor) are retarded on column. Cells able to bind ■ (with ⊏ receptor) pass through.

Inject passed cells into irradiated recipients and challenge with ■ or ▲.

3

Anti- ■ produced

No anti- ▲ produced

Specific binding of lymphocytes to antigen-coated column. [After Wigzell and Makela (1970). *J. Exp. Med.* **132, 110.]**

bound the antigen so that they cannot function as either helper or effector cells. The cells were washed and then injected into lethally irradiated recipients. If thymocytes were the treated cells, a population of normal B-cells was also injected so that T:B cooperation could be tested. Similarly, if B-cells were the treated cells, a population of normal T-cells was injected. The recipients then received two antigens, the specific test antigen and an unrelated one which served as control. It was found that both B-cells and T-cells lost their ability to

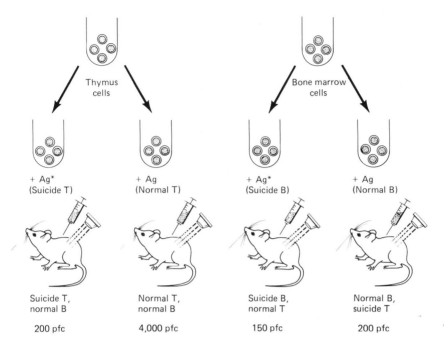

Antigen suicide experiment demonstrating killing of both T-cells and B-cells by high specific activity ^{125}I-labeled antigen (A*). [After Basten et al. (1971). *Nature, New Biol.* **231, 104.]**

participate in antibody formation to the antigen after "suiciding" but made normal responses to the "non-suiciding" antigen. This argues that both effector and helper cells in antibody formation bind antigen specifically.

NATURE OF ANTIGEN-BINDING RECEPTOR

Ig on B-Cells—Possible Receptor Molecules

Since both B-cells and T-cells are able to bind antigen specifically, the next problem is to determine the nature of the receptor which actually binds the antigen. We saw in Chapter 5 that when cell suspensions of mouse lymphoid cells are examined by immuno-fluorescence, some cells have large amounts of surface immunoglobulin. These Ig-positive cells are B-cells. When measured by immunofluorescence methods which are routinely used in immunology studies, spleen has about 65 to 70 percent Ig-positive cells, lymph node about 15 percent but thymus has no Ig-positive cells. The Ig-positive cells are θ negative, which says that T-cells do not have readily detectable amounts of Ig on their surfaces. As a general rule, lymphocytes are Ig^+ θ^- or Ig^- θ^+ (there is a small class of Ig^- θ^- cells called *null cells*).

Since B-cells have easily identifiable surface immunoglobulins, it has been assumed that these immunoglobulin molecules act as receptors for antigen and serve as a means of transmitting a signal to the cell. This would be an economical way for the cell to use its machinery, since the cell would synthesize the same product that is used for recognition. This idea has had some experimental basis. For example, removal of cells on an immunoabsorbent column coated with anti-immunoglobulin results in a loss of function of the passed cells. In other words, a population devoid of Ig-positive cells is nonfunctional. Of course, this is not proof that surface Ig is the antigen-specific receptor since there is the possibility that all B-cells have immunoglobulin on their surface but do not use it as a receptor. If that were the case, the Ig-positive cells would be removed by the reaction with anti-Ig but not because the Ig molecules were acting as receptors.

In Chapter 5, it was pointed out that the Ig on B-cells is predominantly of the IgM and IgD classes with little or no IgG. It has been suggested that the role of IgD may be that of receptor molecule. One of the principle reasons for thinking that IgM or IgD might be the receptor molecule rather than IgG is because so few B-cells have IgG in their surface. In contrast to this notion, it has been hypothesized that a B-cell synthesizes and secretes antibody of the same class that is on its surface. That is, the surface receptor is on a molecule which is the same as the antibody that the cell will synthesize. Because of experimental difficulties, it has been possible to directly test this hypothesis only very recently. The Herzenbergs and their co-workers at Stanford University used a fluorescence-activated cell sorter, a machine which separates cells according to surface markers by allowing a fluorescent labeled antibody to react with the surface antigen, automatically isolating the labeled cells. Their experiment strongly supports the idea that a cell which produces IgG antibody of a certain subclass uses surface IgG of that subclass as its receptor. Mice were primed with an antigen, and cells with IgG on their surface were removed by the cell sorter. These cells were then used to repopulate irradiated recipients. The recipients of the IgG-bearing cells were then challenged with antigen in order to determine what class of Ig the antibody in the secondary response would be. It was found that the majority of antibody-producing cells were producing IgG. In other words, the antibody synthesized in a secondary response was of the same class as the surface Ig on the precursors of the secondary response. This seems to be the strongest evidence to date that the surface Ig of the B-cell is a receptor and that it is a reflection of the synthetic capability of the cell.

Ig on T-cell—A Controversy

Immunoglobulin is easily demonstrated on B-cells but not on T-cells even though functional T-cells bind antigen specifically. If the T-cell does not have immunoglobulin, the question of what mechanism T-cells use to react with antigen must then be answered. Do T-cells have low amounts of Ig on their surface which cannot be detected using ordinary methods; do they have a unique class of Ig on their surface which the anti-immunoglobulin sera used in the fluorescence studies does not detect; or do T-cells bind antigen specifically using receptors which are not immunoglobulin?

The controversy comes from the fact that one research group has been able to demonstrate Ig on the T-cell surface using an iodination method, but several other groups have not been able to reproduce this result. The method in these studies (Figure 5) involves labeling all available tyrosines at the cell surface with radioactive iodine using a lactoperoxidase method. The labeled membrane is then solubilized, and the immunoglobulin which is associated with the membrane is

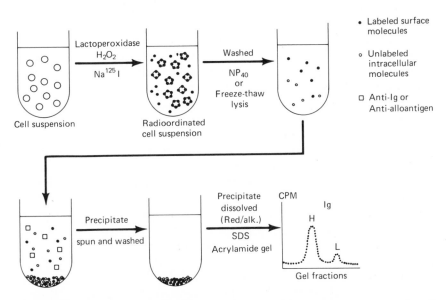

Technique for radioiodination, isolation, and characterization of cell surface molecules from lymphocytes. [After Vitetta *et al.* (1973). *Transplant. Rev.* 14, 50.]

5

precipitated with specific anti-Ig antisera. The specifically precipitated material is then collected and run on disc gel electrophoresis
and analyzed for the presence of radiolabel. When labeled *spleen cells*
are analyzed in this manner, all groups of researchers agree that
membrane-bound Ig is identifiable. This is not surprising since spleen
contains 70 percent B-cells. When either *thymocytes* or *peripheral
T-cells* are analyzed, however, only one group is able to identify
immunoglobulin in the membrane. The others are unable to identify
Ig on T-cell membranes or can account for the small amounts which
they find by nonspecific binding of Ig to the surface. Typical data
from each of these groups is seen in Figure 6. At the moment, the tide
of data seems to be in favor of little or no association of complete Ig
molecules with the T-cell membrane.

Role of H-2 Product as T-Cell Receptor

In Chapter 19 evidence will be presented to show that the genes
which control the antibody responses to a wide variety of antigens are
located in the H-2 complex. There is evidence to show that some of
this H-2 associated genetic control is at the level of antigen recognition by the T-cell. Since, as we have just seen, Ig on T-cells is difficult
to demonstrate, some investigators have argued that recognition of
antigen by the T-cell is not carried out via immunoglobulin
molecules, but rather by a nonimmunoglobulin molecule coded for in
the H-2 region.

This notion of a second set of specific antigen-binding molecules
which are not immunoglobulins has been difficult to test directly.
Very recently, however, data has been generated which allows a
modified form of this theory to be seriously considered. This data
shows that there are some striking structural similarities between
the Ig molecule and the H-2 molecule.

When H-2 or HLA molecules are removed from the membrane of
the cell and analyzed chemically, they are found to have a tetrameric
structure. The tetramer appears to be composed of two large polypeptide chains (called the heavy chains) which contain the H-2 alloan-
tigenic determinants and two smaller chains (the light chains) which
contain a molecule called $\beta2$-*microglobulin*. The $\beta2$-microglobulin
chain is bound to the larger chain by noncovalent interactions, but
the heavy chains are held together by disulfide bonds. It is immediately striking how similar this tetrameric structural arrangement is to that of the immunoglobulin molecule (see Chapter 12).

The similarity between $\beta2$-microglobulin and the immunoglobulin
molecule is taken even further by the fact that when $\beta2$-

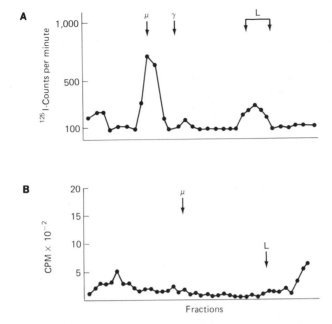

Disc electrophoresis of surface-labeled thymus cells. In (A) immuno-globulin is found. In (B) no immunoglobulin is found. [A after Mar-chelonis and Cone (1973). *Transplant. Rev.* **14, 3. B after Vitetta** *et al.* **(1972).** *J. Exp. Med.* **136, 81.]**

6

microglobulin molecules are sequenced, great sequence homology (see Chapter 14) is found between the β2-microglobulin and a portion of the Ig heavy chain. This argues for potential common ancestry of the genes. Furthermore, there are intrachain disulfide bonds and chain loops in the H-2 heavy chain which are analogous to those which define the structural domains of the Ig heavy chain. *Staph A protein,* a material which binds preferentially to the Fc region of immuno-globulin molecules, also binds to the H-2 and HLA heavy chains. Considering all these facts together shows that there is a molecular complex at the cell surface with structural similarity to Ig but which is coded for in part by H-2. This molecule is a current strong candidate for the T-cell antigen receptor molecule, although still unanswered is the crucial question of where on the molecule the specificity sequences are to be found. This question is addressed in the idiotype experiments covered below.

Common Idiotypic Determinants on T- and B-Cells

Whatever the chemical nature of the receptors on B- and T-cells, a recent elegant piece of work shows that both of these cell types share idiotypes at their surface. It will be seen in Chapter 13 that an idiotype is a unique antigen-binding site on an antibody molecule. The antibody molecules directed against a certain antigen will have an area in the region of the molecule that binds antigen which is itself uniquely antigenic. Taking advantage of this fact, it is possible to make antibodies which are directed against the antigen-binding sites of other antibody molecules. It has been possible to show that such a region which is specific for a certain antigen appears on both T- and B-cell surfaces. Presumably this is a molecule which the cell could use to recognize antigen. As we will see, the exact chemical nature of the molecule is not yet known, but the binding site is one shared with immunoglobulin. It has been postulated that this small portion of an immunoglobulin molecule (the combining site) attached to the H-2:β2-microglobulin complex may confer antigen specificity.

To demonstrate an idiotypic determinant, one must generate an antibody against it. The method to produce the anti-idiotype antisera used by Wigzell in his studies takes advantage of the fact that parental cells injected into an F_1 are not recognized as foreign but are able to recognize antigens on the F_1 cells. This was the basis for the GVH reaction (Chapter 4). Now, if the parental cells are able to recognize an antigen on the F_1 cells, they must have cell surface receptors for that antigen. The F_1 does not react against itself, so it does not have the receptor. Therefore, the F_1, while not recognizing any histocompatability antigens on the parental cells, should recognize as foreign the *antigen-binding receptors* which the parental strain uses to recognize antigens on the F_1 and produce antibodies against them. If the receptor is immunoglobulin, the antibody directed against the combining site will be an anti-idiotype antibody.

In this situation, the F_1 produced antibody against a receptor molecule on one of the parental cells. The receptor was the receptor for antigen on the cells of the other parent (i.e., an anti-receptor antibody was produced). In other words, one parent has antigen A and the other antigen B, so that the F_1 has both A and B. The parent with A antigens has receptors for B antigens, and this is the determinant which the anti-idiotype antibody is directed against. By adding complement to the anti-idiotype-cell complex, all the cells in the A parent which have receptors that are directed against antigens on the B parent should be lysed. If they are lysed, the remaining cells should not be able to generate a cell-mediated response against the cells of parent B. This was exactly the result obtained. After reacting with the anti-idiotype which is directed against receptors for antigen B on A cells, the A cells could not react against cells of parent B but were able to react against strain C (an unrelated strain). The anti-idiotype antibodies have been shown to react with both B-cells and T-cells. The idiotype determinant has recently been shown to be linked to the H chains of immunoglobulins and not the L chains (see Chapter 13 for details of H and L chains).

This incredibly complex experiment is one of the first break-throughs leading to identification of part of an immunoglobulin molecule being part of the T-cell receptor. It could also explain why the T-cell Ig has been so elusive. Several investigators have tenta-tively proposed that the V region of the immunoglobulin molecule (the idiotypic determinant) may be chemically combined with the H-2 in the membrane. If this is so, it could account for the association of H-2 and T-cell recognition.

NATURE OF THE SIGNAL

One Signal vs. Two Signals

Up to now we have established that both B- and T-cells specifi-cally bind antigen at their surface, although the chemical nature of the receptor responsible for this binding on the T-cell is not known. We know that receptors on both B-cells and T-cells contain idiotypic markers. We will see in Chapter 17 that antigen induces lymphocytes to proliferate and differentiate, causing the specific expansion of reactive clones which is the central idea of a clonal selection mechanism. Another great unanswered question is the nature of the "signal" to the lymphocytes which is brought about by the interaction of the surface receptor and antigen.

In both antibody and cell-mediated responses, the response of the effector cell precursor to antigen requires some sort of interaction from the helper cell for the functional effector cell to be generated. In a *two-signal model* the interaction of the surface receptor on the effector cell precursor with antigen is considered the first signal. The helper cell is thought to supply the second signal as a soluble factor or by cell contact. A single signal will not lead to effector cell function. One version of a two-signal model has the first signal in the absence of the second leading to tolerance. In a *one-signal model* the interac-tion of antigen and receptor is sufficient for the effector cell precursor to become a functional effector cell. Since effector-helper interaction in cell-mediated responses has been discovered only recently, more work and thought has gone into the problem of one or two signals in antibody formation than in cell-mediated responses.

Two-Signal Models

Some of the most elaborate model building in recent years has been done in association with one or two signals. Experiments are difficult to perform in this area because we do not know the nature of the receptors or the signals. But the kind of experiment which would argue for two signals would be to deliver the first signal to cells in the absence of the second signal to see if the first signal would induce some change in the cells. Such an experiment, which shows that contact with antigen in the absence of T-cells can lead to proliferation of B-cells but not their differentiation into antibody-producing cells, is seen in Figure 7. In the experiment, the spleens of *nude* mice were the source of B-cells. The nude mouse is a congenitally athymic mutant. Since it has no thymus it is a substitute for either neonatal thymectomy or anti-θ treated cells. These B-cells were cultured with antigen for 40 hr in the absence of T-cells, and then T-cells were added as the second signal. In one experimental group a block to mitosis was added 27 hr after antigen. This experiment asks two questions: Can antibody be produced by B-cells if helper cells are added 40 hr later, and, if it can, does the clonal expansion of the B-cells which is due to proliferation occur before or after the addition of T-cell help; i.e., was there proliferation in response to antigen in the absence of T-cell help (signal 1) and differentiation into antibody-forming cells when T-cell help was provided (signal 2)?

With no addition of T-cell help there was no antibody production (as expected), but when helper T-cells were added 40 hr after antigen, the B-cells did give rise to antibody-forming cells. In the group in which the block of proliferation in response to antigen was added at 27 hr, there was no antibody production when T-cells were added. This experiment can therefore be interpreted as showing that antigen induces proliferation of B-cell precursor cells in the absence of T-cell help, but the T-cell is required to allow the cells which have proliferated to differentiate into antibody-producing cells. Stated in terms of signal theory, the antigen provides signal one, and the T-cell or its product provides signal two.

One-Signal Model Based on Mitogenicity

We saw in Chapter 5 that some mitogens are specific for T-cells (PHA, ConA) and some for B-cells (pokeweed, LPS). If LPS is added to a culture of mouse spleen cells under appropriate conditions, a small but definite number of antibody-forming cells are generated against a wide variety of antigens even though the antigen has not been added to the culture. This is probably due to the nonspecific activation by mitogen of B-cell clones which are programmed to respond to the

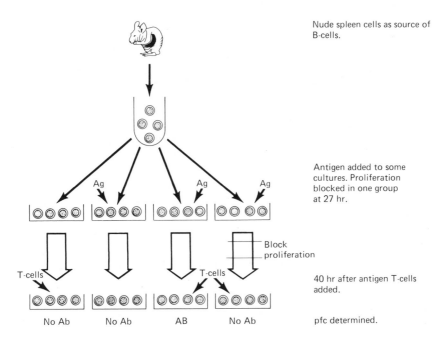

Nude spleen cells as source of B-cells.

Antigen added to some cultures. Proliferation blocked in one group at 27 hr.

Block proliferation

40 hr after antigen T-cells added.

pfc determined.

7

Experiment dividing antigen (signal 1) and T-cell help (signal 2). [After Dutton (1975). *Transplant. Rev.* 23, 66.]

antigens. This kind of activation of B-cell clones is called POLYCLONAL ACTIVATION. As a general rule, T-independent antigens act as B-cell mitogens. Putting these two facts together, Möller and Coutinho have generated a rather appealing theory which argues that T-independent antigens have *inherent mitogenicity* and this mitogenicity is the signal to the B-cell. The theory argues that T-independent antigens have a full measure of "inherent mitogenicity" but that T-dependent antigens need help from the T-cell to get full mitogenicity. In this model the role of the surface Ig on the B-cell surface is not as a signal generator, but rather merely as a means of *focusing* antigen onto the surface of the cell so that the mitogenic part of the antigen can then react with some unknown mitogen-receptor. In this manner the signal to the cell is generated by the mitogen. In this model the role of the antigen receptor is only to bring the proper concentration of mitogen onto the cell surface. Most antigens require help from T-cells to give the full mitogenic stimulus.

A strong point in favor of this theory comes from the fact that one strain of mouse, C3H/He, has B-cells which are refractory to the mitogenic action of LPS. When hapten is conjugated to LPS, it acts as a thymus-independent antigen in all strains except C3H/He. Thus, in the one strain unable to respond to this B-cell mitogen, there is no antibody formation to a hapten coupled to the mitogen. The simplest forms of the signal models are diagrammed in Figure 8.

MEMBRANE REORGANIZATION AND SIGNALS

During the past several years the conception of the molecular organization of the membrane of cells has changed largely through studies done on lymphocytes. The traditional view of the cell membrane of all cells had been one of a rigid molecular bilayer of protein and lipid. Frye and Edidin in 1970 questioned this view of the membrane on the basis of work they had done in which cells with different H-2 antigens were fused and the redistribution of the H-2 molecules in the membrane studied. They saw that there was a rapid redistribution of H-2 molecules so that the fused cells soon had a uniform distribution of both sets of H-2 molecules on their surfaces. As a reason for this they proposed that there were large areas of membrane which were fluid rather than rigid.

Patching and Capping

The conclusion that the membrane may be fluid was supported by work on lymphocytes in which it was possible to show that various antigens on the surface of lymphocytes could move in the plane of the membrane if they were reacted with an appropriate antibody. Experimentally, fluorescein-labeled anti-Ig is added to lymphocytes, and the pattern of fluorescence on the surface of B-cells is examined at short intervals of time. Immediately after adding the labeled anti-Ig there is a ring pattern of fluorescence around the surface of the Ig-positive cells. This indicates that the Ig molecules on the B-cells are arranged all around the cell, probably in a random fashion. This is seen in Figure 9. Very soon, however, the ring pattern of fluorescence changes and patches of label are seen. After a short time the patches of label all move to one pole of the cell, forming a cap. This process is called PATCHING and CAPPING. Very often the capped material is ingested by the cell by pinocytosis.

Significance

It has been argued by some that the signal to the cell is the result of molecular reorganization of the membrane after reaction with antigen. This is an appealing notion which can be tested experimen-

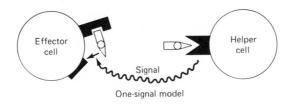

One-signal model

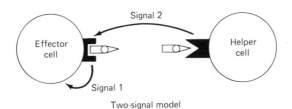

Two-signal model

8

One- and two-signal models for effector cell activation.

tally; however, there is no compelling reason at the moment to accept or reject the idea.

IMMUNE RECOGNITION BY ALTERED SELF

In this chapter attention has been directed to the nature of the receptor which the lymphocyte uses to recognize and react with antigen. Very recently, experiments have been reported which may have bearing on the orientation of antigen which allows the receptors

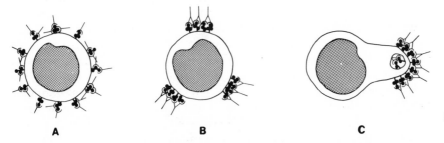

A   B   C

9

Patching and capping of surface Ig on lymphocytes. (A) Uniform distribution of Ig molecules. (B) Anti-Ig causes patches of membrane Ig molecules. (C) Surface Ig molecules cap at one end of the cell. [After Taylor et al. (1971). Nature, New Biol. 233, 225.]

on the lymphocytes to react properly. The experiments so far all involve T-cell effector cells in cytotoxic responses to several antigens, but they may be pointing to the mechanism by which T-cells recognize all foreign material.

The basic experiment is seen in Figure 10. Mice were immunized to antigen such as certain viruses, TNP, or some non-H-2 tissue antigen. Spleen cells of these mice were then cultured on antigen-coated ^{51}Cr labeled fibroblasts which serve as target cells for a standard CML assay. If the immunized mice are H-2^k when the antigen is coated on H-2^k target cells, there is killing of the target cells. However when the antigen-coated targets are of another H-2 haplotype, for example, H-2^d or H-2^b, there is no killing by the H-2^k effector cells. If the effector cells were from H-2^d mice, they could kill only coated target cells from an H-2^d mice and not labeled cells from mice of other haplotypes. This very important observation, originally made by Zinkernagel and Doherty, has been interpreted as showing that the effector cell in CML must *recognize altered self* to carry out its killing.

By the proper use of recombinants it has been shown that there must be identity at the K or D ends of the H-2 complex between labeled monolayer and reactive T-cell. This means that virus or some other antigen which is bound to molecules at the K or D regions of the H-2 complex of the animal's own haplotype are recognized as foreign but not those bound to the K or D molecules of another haplotype.

This very provocative discovery has led to the concept of recognition of *altered self*. In this notion, antigen reacts with H-2 molecules on the cells of the animal. T-cells of the responding animal recognize the antigen only when it is associated with its own H-2 molecules which have been slightly altered by the antigen since the responding cells do not react with cells not coated with antigen. If, as clonal selection implies, reactions are carried out by lymphocytes already committed to reacting with certain antigens, then we must begin to consider the possibility that the lymphocytes are committed to react with slightly altered forms of "self." This would make sense if a major function of the immune response is surveillance against new antigens, e.g., tumor antigens which may be slightly altered forms of self. It might also explain why normal animals have so many functional cells directed against H-2 antigens.

An alternative interpretation is one of *dual recognition*. In this explanation it is postulated that the hapten or virus is recognized and at the same time the unaltered H-2 molecule is also recognized. This

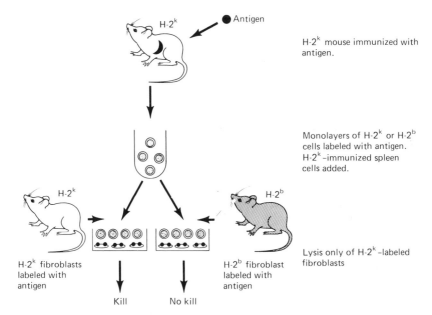

Antigen recognition by altered self. [After Zinkernagel and Doherty (1974). *Nature* **248, 701.]**

10

means that controlled autoreactivity would be part of T-cell responses.

The implications of this concept are so far-reaching that these kinds of experiments and the exploration of this notion will most likely become a major area of investigation in the next several years. An added philosophical turn here is the idea that H-2 may be acting as an integral part of both the antigen which is reacted against and the receptor molecule which does the reacting. One of the many unanswered questions in immunology has been why there are so many cells reactive to H-2 alloantigens. If these cells are part of the repertoire of cells reactive to both self and altered self, this would account for their great number.

SUMMARY

1. The number of precursors of antibody-forming cells is determined by the focus-forming cell assay. There is 1 antigen-specific reactive antibody-forming precursor cell per 10^{-6} cells.

2. There are 100 to 1,000 times more cells reactive to an antigen when measured by the binding of labeled antigen to cells.

3. There are very high numbers of cells reactive in GVH.

4. Functional B-cells and T-cells both bind antigen specifically.

5. The chemical nature of the surface receptor for antigen binding is not known, but it is generally agreed that immunoglobulin is the likely candidate for B-cells. There is controversy about the presence ᶠ Ig in the membranes of T-cells. Most investigators are unable to aᴜmonstrate T-cell surface Ig.

6. Products of the H-2 region may be associated with the T-cell receptor. There is a structural analogy between H-2 and Ig.

7. Both B-cells and T-cells have idiotype determinants on their surfaces. It is possible that this small portion of an Ig may be associated with the H-2 product and serve as the T-cell receptor.

8. The nature of the signal which interaction with a surface receptor imparts to the lymphocyte is not known. It has been postulated that antigen acts as one signal but a second signal from the T-cell is needed by B-cells. Another theory postulates that a single signal based on mitogenicity is sufficient to trigger a B-cell.

9. Antigen can induce reorganization of membrane molecules (such as receptors), and this reorganization in the form of patching and capping may be part of the signal.

10. Recognition of antigen may be due in part to antigen combination with H-2 products and the recognition of these products as altered self.

READINGS

REVIEWS

Warner, N. L. (1974). Membrane immunoglobulins and antigen receptors on B and T-lymphocytes, *Adv. Immunol.* **19,** 67.

Ada, G. L. (1970). Antigen binding cells in tolerance and immunity, *Transplant. Rev.* **5,** 105.

Davie, J. M., and Paul, W. E. (1974). Antigen binding receptors on lymphocytes, *Contemp. Top. Immunobiol.* **3,** 171.

(Three reviews covering Ig on cells and their possible role as receptors.)

Bretscher, P. A., and Cohn, M. (1968). Minimal model for the mechanism of antibody induction and paralysis by antigen, *Nature,* **220,** 444. (The two signal model.)

Coutinho, A., and Möller, G. (1975). Thymus-independent B-cell induction and paralysis, *Adv. Immunol.* **21,** 114. (The arguments in favor of the one signal model.)

ARTICLES

Marchalonis, J. J., Cone, R. E., and Atwell, J. L. (1972). Isolation and partial characterization of lymphocyte surface immunoglobulins, *J. Exp. Med.* **135,** 956.

Vitetta, E. S., Bianco, C., Nussenzweig, V., and Uhr, J. W. (1972). Cell surface immunoglobulin. IV. Distribution among thymocytes, bone marrow cells, and their derived populations, *J. Exp. Med.* **136,** 81. (The principal participants in the T-cell Ig controversy.)

Binz, H., and Wigzell, H. (1975). Shared idiotypic determinants on B and T lymphocytes reactive against the same antigenic determinants. I. Demonstration of similar or identical idiotypes of IgG molecules and T-cell receptors with specificity for the same alloantigens, *J. Exp. Med.* **142,** 197.

—— and —— (1975). Shared idiotypic determinants on B and T lymphocytes reactive against the same antigenic determinants. III. Physical fractionation of specific immunocompetent T lymphocytes by affinity chromatography using anti-idiotypic antibodies. *J. Exp. Med.* **142,** 1231.

Wigzell, H. (1976). Inheritance of T-cell receptors specific for transplantation antigens is linked to the genes coding for the heavy chains of immunoglobulins. *Cold Spring Harbor Symposium on Quant. Biol.,* in press.

Zinkernagel, R. M., and Doherty, P. C. (1975). H-2 compatability requirement for T-cell-mediated lysis of target cells infected with lymphocytic choriomeningitis virus, *J. Exp. Med.* **141,** 1427. (The altered-self concept.)

11

ROLE OF THE MACROPHAGE

OVERVIEW

In the last several chapters we have been building up the argument that specificity in the immune response is brought about by lymphocytes which react specifically with antigen by means of antigen-specific receptors at the cell surface. The macrophage is a cell essential to the functioning of lymphocytes but which is not antigen specific. Antibody responses, cell-mediated responses, and mitogen responses all require the presence of the macrophage. The macrophage, therefore, is one of the three important cell types in the immune response. In this chapter we will try to define the role and function of macrophages in the immune response.

NEED FOR MACROPHAGES IN IMMUNE RESPONSES

Macrophages are usually defined as large mononuclear, phagocytic cells which adhere to glass or plastic surfaces. They are found fixed in tissues (e.g., spleen, Kupffer cells in liver, or dendritic cells in lymph nodes) or free in peritoneal exudates and the circulation. Peritoneal exudate is an especially rich source of macrophages.

Antibody Production in Vivo

A typical experiment which shows that macrophages are necessary for antibody production *in vivo* is outlined in Figure 1. If an animal is given a nonlethal dose of X-irradiation, its spleen is

146

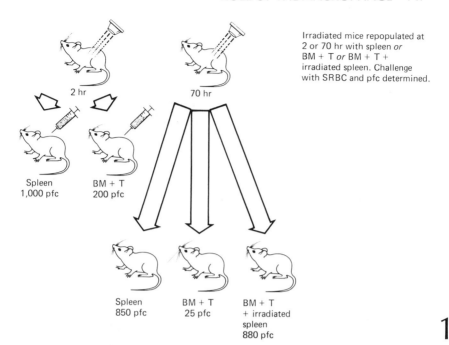

Irradiated mice repopulated at 2 or 70 hr with spleen *or* BM + T *or* BM + T + irradiated spleen. Challenge with SRBC and pfc determined.

2 hr   70 hr

Spleen   BM + T
1,000 pfc   200 pfc

Spleen   BM + T   BM + T
850 pfc   25 pfc   + irradiated
                        spleen
                        880 pfc

1

Effect of delay after X-ray on reconstitution of antibody response showing that radiation-resistant macrophages leave the spleen by 70 hr. [From Gorczynski *et al.* (1971). *J. Exp. Med.* 134, 1201.]

depleted of macrophages 70 hr later. If the macrophage is involved in antibody formation, these mice with no splenic macrophages should not make antibody when repopulated with bone marrow and thymus cells. Repopulation with spleen cells, however, should allow antibody to be formed since spleen cells will contain B-cell, T-cells, and macrophages. In the experiment in Figure 1, lethally irradiated mice were injected with either spleen cells or bone marrow plus thymus cells within 2 hr after irradiation when macrophages were still present in the spleen or after a delay of 70 hr following irradiation when macrophages were not present. All the groups were challenged with antigen at the time of repopulation. It was found that in recipients repopulated immediately after X-ray, good antibody responses were obtained in mice repopulated with either spleen cells alone or bone marrow plus thymus. However, waiting 70 hr after X-ray to repopulate the mice led to antibody responses only in mice repopulated with spleen cells but not in those repopulated with bone marrow plus thymus. Injection of spleen cells which had been irradiated along with bone marrow and thymus in the 70-hr group allowed the marrow-thymus cooperation to occur.

The two conclusions to be drawn from these data are first, that bone marrow and thymus cells cannot cooperate in mice when the macrophages have left the spleen and, second, that the addition of freshly irradiated spleen replaces these cells, which shows that the function of the macrophages is radiation-resistant.

Antibody Production in Vitro

An experiment demonstrating the need for the macrophage in generating an antibody response *in vitro* was seen in the experiment in Figure 3 in Chapter 3 in which spleen cells were separated into nonadhering (NA) and adhering (A) populations. The NA cells were lymphocyte-rich, and the A cells were macrophage-rich by morphological criteria. Neither NA nor A populations produced antibody to SRBC when cultured alone, but when the two populations were combined, they were able to produce antibody. The B-cells in the NA population produced the antibody using the T-cells in the NA population as a source of helper cells, but the macrophage population (the A population) was required for this cooperation to occur. Macrophage involvement is a general rule for responses to thymus-dependent antigens. The need for macrophages in responses to thymus-independent antigens is open to question.

Cell-Mediated Responses.

Macrophages are also required to generate cytotoxic cells in a CML response. In the experiment shown in Figure 2, CBA (H-2^k) cells were immunized against BALB/c (H-2^d) cells in the presence or absence of macrophages. Cytotoxic effector activity of the CBA cells was determined by ^{51}Cr release from DBA/2 target cells. It can be seen that in the absence of macrophages the numbers of cytotoxic cells generated were greatly reduced.

Proliferative Responses

The data in Table 1 shows that macrophages must be present in cultures to which the mitogens PHA or ConA have been added for a proliferative response to occur to these mitogens. It can be seen that with T-cells alone, in the absence of macrophages, there is a poor proliferative response to either mitogen. The addition of macrophages to the cultures, however, results in generation of the responses to control levels.

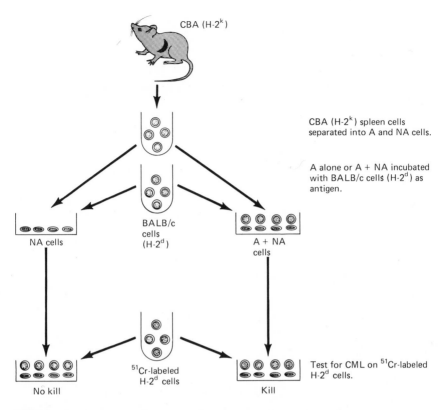

CBA (H-2^k) spleen cells separated into A and NA cells.

A alone or A + NA incubated with BALB/c cells (H-2^d) as antigen.

NA cells

BALB/c cells (H-2^d)

A + NA cells

No kill

^{51}Cr-labeled H-2^d cells

Kill

Test for CML on ^{51}Cr-labeled H-2^d cells.

2

Effect of presence of macrophages on generation of CML effector cells. [From Wagner *et al.* (1972). *J. Exp. Med.* **136**, 331.]

TABLE 1.   NEED FOR MACROPHAGES IN PROLIFERATIVE RESPONSES TO MITOGENS.

	^{3}H incorporation (cpm)		
	No mitogen	*ConA*	*PHA*
T lymphocytes alone	94	233	412
T lymphocytes + macrophages	279	5,900	55,200

From Rosenstreich *et al.* (1976). *J. Immunol.* **116**, 131.

Macrophages as Accessory Cells

Not all cells meeting the physical criteria of macrophages serve as cells able to function in the immune response, as demonstrated in the following experiment. If bone marrow is cultured under appropriate *in vitro* conditions, large, adherent, mononuclear, phagocytic cells are present in large numbers in the culture after a few days. Even though they meet the physical criteria of macrophages, these cells are not able to cooperate with B- and T-cells in generating an *in vitro* antibody response. They cannot replace the adherent cell obtained from spleen or the cell from the peritoneal exudate. Because of this we can conclude that only certain cells meeting the morphological criteria of macrophages can function in the immune response. These cells are often called ACCESSORY CELLS. In this chapter we will use the terms *macrophage* and *accessory cell* interchangeably, but it should be kept in mind that we are interested only in the macrophages which aid in carrying out immune function.

FUNCTIONS OF MACROPHAGES IN ANTIBODY RESPONSES

The role which the macrophage plays in the generation of antibody has been more extensively studied than its role in cell-mediated responses, but still the precise mechanism of its function is not known. We will discuss several of the current ideas concerning the possible function of macrophages in antibody responses. As we go on, it will be seen that even though the experiments designed to test the function of the macrophage are internally consistent, they are either not measuring a phenomenon of biological significance or there are several means by which macrophages carry out their function. Broadly speaking the four proposed possible mechanisms of macrophage function in antibody production are:

1. Antigen processing for presentation to lymphocytes
2. Antigen processing by elaboration of soluble factors
3. Providing nutritional factors
4. Information transfer

All or any of these could also play a role in cell-mediated responses.

Antigen Processing and Direct Presentation

The basis of this idea is that the function of the macrophage is to somehow put antigen into a suitable immunogenic form. Imagine a red blood cell or large molecule with multiple antigenic determinants; a possible role of the macrophage would be to somehow break the antigen down to proper size (or form) and then present it to the lymphocyte so that the lymphocyte can respond to the appropriate determinant. Presentation could involve proper configuration for cross-linking receptors, antigen focusing, or other means of allowing antigen to react properly with a lymphocyte.

Part of the experimental justification of this notion comes from the fact that antigen which is associated with macrophages is more immunogenic than antigen not associated with macrophages. The experiment shown in Figure 3 demonstrates this point. Radioactive labeled antigen was injected into mice, and then the peritoneal macrophages which had phagocytized the antigen were harvested. Because the antigen was labeled, determining the amount of antigen which was associated with the macrophages was possible. Varying numbers of these macrophages with associated antigen (macrophage-associated antigen) were then injected into normal nonirradiated mice. Other groups of mice were injected with the same concentration of antigen which was not macrophage-associated. In this manner it

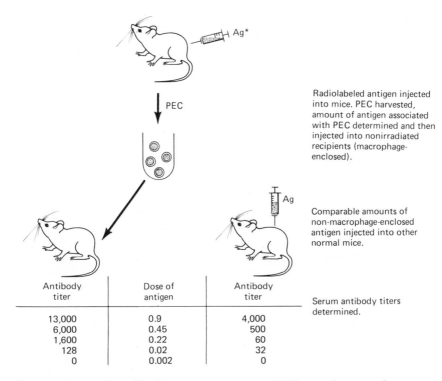

Radiolabeled antigen injected into mice. PEC harvested, amount of antigen associated with PEC determined and then injected into nonirradiated recipients (macrophage-enclosed).

Comparable amounts of non-macrophage-enclosed antigen injected into other normal mice.

Serum antibody titers determined.

Antibody titer	Dose of antigen	Antibody titer
13,000	0.9	4,000
6,000	0.45	500
1,600	0.22	60
128	0.02	32
0	0.002	0

3

Comparison of antibody responses to soluble antigen and macrophage-enclosed antigen. [From Unanue and Askonas (1968). *Immunology*, 15, 287.]

was possible to measure the effect of the macrophage on the immunogenicity of the antigen. It was found that more antibody was produced in response to a given amount of macrophage-associated antigen than to a comparable amount of soluble antigen.

It has been found that the vast majority of antigen taken up by macrophages is catabolized after 24 hr. However, a small amount of antigen remains at the surface of the macrophage. Removal of this material with proteolytic enzymes eliminates the ability of the macrophage to give enhanced immunogenicity. This is interpreted as showing that *surface bound* macrophage-associated antigen is the antigen which is effective in an experiment such as the one illustrated in Figure 3.

Another model which involves antigen presentation via the macrophage was seen in Chapter 9. In this model the T-cell immunoglobulin (Ig-T) reacted with antigen, and the Ig-T-antigen complex was thought to be shed and to become associated with the surface of the macrophage. The macrophage Ig-T-antigen complex then comes in contact with the B-cell to give the complete signal to the B-cell.

Antigen Processing by Elaboration of Soluble Factors

Another mechanism of macrophage function could be the processing of antigen by *soluble factors*. An experiment which argues in favor of this model is diagrammed in Figure 4. In this experiment a macrophage-rich cell suspension was cultured with SRBC antigen (group B), and the supernate of this culture was then added to a culture of lymphocytes from which the macrophages had been removed (macrophage-depleted spleen cells). The lymphocytes produced antibody when the supernate was added but not in the absence of the supernate. There was no further addition of antigen, so this argues that the supernate contained immunogenic antigen which the macrophages had processed.

When macrophages were incubated in the *absence* of SRBC (group C), and the supernatant of this culture was added to macrophage-depleted spleen cells to which SRBC were added, the lymphocytes were able to produce antibody. This argues that the supernate of the macrophage culture is able to substitute for macrophages in the final culture. When macrophages were incubated alone, then supernatant removed and the supernate incubated overnight with SRBC and the SRBC removed (group D), it was found that the resulting supernate still substitutes for macrophages and antigen. All these findings can be most easily interpreted as showing that macrophages produce a soluble factor which acts as an antigen processor and that the processed antigen is immunogenic.

A

pfc
20

Lymphocytes
+ RBC

Lymphocytes in absence of
macrophages give low pfc
response.

B
Supernate

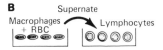

Macrophages
+ RBC   Lymphocytes

148

Macrophages incubated with
RBC. Supernate added to
lymphocytes restores response.

C
Supernate

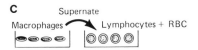

Macrophages   Lymphocytes + RBC

210

Macrophages incubated without
RBC. Supernate added to
lymphocytes + RBC restores
response.

D
Supernate   Supernate

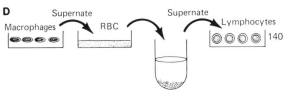

Macrophages   RBC   Lymphocytes

140

Macrophages incubated without
RBC. RBC added to supernate.
RBC removed and supernate
added to lymphocytes.
Response restored.

4

**Activity of macrophage supernates in antigen processing. [After
Shortman and Palmer (1971).** *Cell. Immunol.* **2, 399.]**

Nutritional Factors

There is data which shows that the macrophage may play a
"nutritional" role rather than an antigen-processing role in the initiation of *in vitro* antibody responses. In fact, the simple chemical
2-*mercaptoethanol* can be shown to substitute for macrophages. In the
experiment shown in Figure 5 spleen populations were depleted of
macrophages and cultured in the Mishell-Dutton *in vitro* system. The
nonadherent cells failed to make antibody (as expected), but when
mercaptoethanol was added to the macrophage-depleted cell suspension, the ability to generate antibody production was restored. It is
generally felt that mercaptoethanol acts in a manner which improves
culture conditions, perhaps by neutralizing toxic cell products,
thereby allowing the lymphocytes to function.

Transfer of Genetic Information

Incubating normal lymphocytes with phenol extracts of immune
peritoneal exudate cells (PEC) *in vitro* results in antibody production

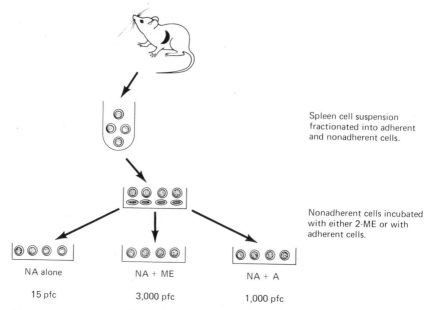

Spleen cell suspension
fractionated into adherent
and nonadherent cells.

Nonadherent cells incubated
with either 2-ME or with
adherent cells.

NA alone

15 pfc

NA + ME

3,000 pfc

NA + A

1,000 pfc

5

Mercaptoethanol (ME) replaces adherent cells in antibody production.
[After Chen and Hirsch (1972). *J. Exp. Med.* 136, 604.]

by the normal lymphocytes. The material from the PEC responsible
for the conversion of normal cells to immune cells appears to be RNA.
Antigen has been found to be associated with some of the RNA
extracted from PEC, and this antigen-RNA complex seems to be
responsible for some antibody production, but a lighter RNA fraction
which has no detectable antigen associated with it is responsible for a
good proportion of the antibody produced. This RNA has been termed
"immune RNA."

By using as donors of the "immune RNA" rabbits or mice with
allotype markers different from those of the animals used as donors of
the responding lymphocytes, it has been possible to design experiments which begin to test if the antigen-free extract is acting as a
transmitter of genetic information.[1] When the cells from which the
RNA is extracted come from a homozygous *a* allotype animal and the
normal lymphocytes come from a homozygous *b* allotype animal, it is
possible to tell if the lymphocytes are making antibody of their own

[1]See Chapter 13 for details of allotypes. For the present it is sufficient to know that
an allotype is a genetically determined antigen on an immunoglobulin molecule.

allotype or of the allotype of the RNA donor. If the lymphocytes from the allotype *b* animal produce antibody which has the *a* allotype, this can be interpreted as showing that somehow the RNA has converted the lymphocytes into cells able to synthesize immunoglobulin of an allotype which they have no genes to produce. This kind of result has been obtained by workers in at least one laboratory. Before sweeping conclusions can be drawn about the role of genetic information transfer in immune responses, this very provocative and important observation must be confirmed and the "immune RNA" subjected to intense chemical analysis.

ARMED AND ACTIVATED MACROPHAGES

As well as acting as an accessory cell in the generation of antibody and cell-mediated responses, the macrophage can function as an effector cell against tumors or allogeneic cells and as a cell which destroys invading bacteria.

Armed Macrophages

Under certain experimental conditions the macrophage can act as a specific cytotoxic cell for tumors. These macrophages are called "armed" macrophages. We saw that in its role as an accessory cell the macrophage had no specificity. In its role as an effector cell, it derives its specificity from molecules liberated by lymphocytes. These molecules become attached to the macrophage surface, hence the notion of the macrophage being "armed."

The experimental system which shows the arming of macrophages is illustrated in Figure 6. Macrophages were removed from the peritoneal cavity of CBA mice which had been immunized against a lymphoma (lymphoid tumor) from C57BL/6 mice. The macrophages were cultured *in vitro* as a monolayer. When C57BL/6 lymphoma cells were added to the culture, they were killed by the monolayer cells. The macrophages from mice immunized against the C57BL/6 lymphoma killed 99 percent of the lymphoma cells derived from C57BL/6 but less than 10 percent of lymphoma cells from DBA/2. If the mice had been immunized to the DBA/2 lymphoma, there would have been killing of only the DBA/2 cells and not the C57BL/6 lymphoma cells. Similarly, if the mice had been immunized with a bacterial metabolic product elaborated into the culture medium called PPD, the macrophages killed neither the C57BL/6 nor the DBA/2 lymphoma cells. We thus have an example of specific effector function by macrophages.

Specific killing of lymphoma cells by macrophages. [After Evans and Alexander (1972). *Nature* 236, 168.]

Arming by the T-Cell

The specificity for the killing of the lymphoma cells by the macrophages of the immunized mice is conferred upon the macrophages by the T-cells of the immunized mice. To show this, CBA mice were immunized with DBA/2 lymphoma, and the spleen cells were cultured *in vitro* in the presence of killed DBA/2 lymphoma cells. After 24 hr the supernate was removed and added to a *normal* macrophage monolayer. When viable DBA/2 lymphoma cells were added, they were killed. We thus have a situation in which immunized spleen cells liberate a product which confers the ability to kill lymphoma cells upon the macrophages; i.e., they have "armed" the normal macrophages. If the spleen cells were treated with anti-θ and complement before they were incubated with the killed lymphoma, no factor was elaborated and the macrophages were not armed. This shows that the soluble factor which arms the macrophage is a product of the T-cell.

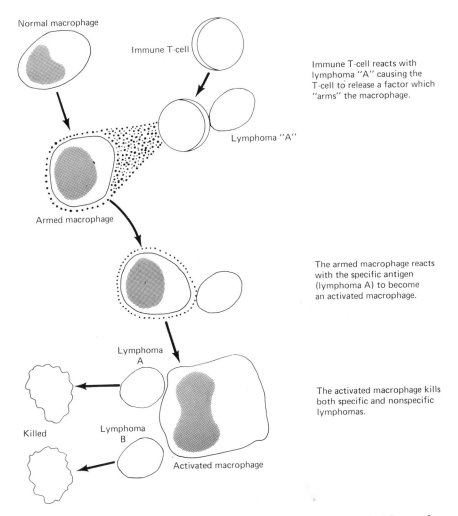

Normal macrophage

Immune T-cell

Immune T-cell reacts with lymphoma "A" causing the T-cell to release a factor which "arms" the macrophage.

Lymphoma "A"

Armed macrophage

The armed macrophage reacts with the specific antigen (lymphoma A) to become an activated macrophage.

Lymphoma A

The activated macrophage kills both specific and nonspecific lymphomas.

Killed

Lymphoma B

Activated macrophage

7

Armed and activated macrophages. [After Evans and Alexander (1972). *Nature* **236, 168.]**

Activated Macrophages

   The "activated" macrophage is a macrophage which has enhanced ability to carry out a macrophage function. Experiments with "armed" macrophages have shown that once armed and having reacted with the specific antigen, the macrophage becomes activated and can then kill nonspecifically. In other words, the macrophage must be "armed," and the arming is specific. Once armed with the

T-cell product, it is able to react with the specific antigen. This specific reaction "activates" the macrophage, but the activated macrophage kills nonspecifically. This is shown diagrammatically in Figure 7.

SUMMARY

1. Macrophages are large mononuclear, phagocytic cells which adhere to glass or plastic surfaces.
2. Macrophages are required for antibody production, the generation of cell-mediated responses, and mitogenic responses. They do not have antigen specificity.
3. The function of the macrophage is not known. Possible modes of function are by antigen processing, elaboration of soluble factors, nutritional factors, or information transfer.
4. The "armed" macrophage is a macrophage which has acquired antigenic specificity from a T-cell product. "Armed" macrophages can destroy target cells. An "armed" macrophage, after reacting with its specific antigen, becomes "activated." An "activated" macrophage kills nonspecifically.

READINGS

REVIEW

Unanue, E. R. (1972). The regulatory role of macrophages in antigenic stimulation, *Adv. Immunol.* **15**, 95.

ARTICLES

Mosier, D. E. (1967). A requirement for two cell types for antibody formation *in vitro, Science,* **158**, 1575.

Rosenstreich, D. L., Farrar, J. J., and Dougherty, S. (1976). Absolute macrophage dependency of T lymphocyte activation by mitogens, *J. Immunol.* **116**, 131.

Wagner, H., Feldmann, M., Boyle, W., and Schrader, J. W. (1972). Cell-mediated immune response *in vitro*. III. Requirement for macrophages in cytotoxic reactions against cell-bound and subcellular alloantigens, *J. Exp. Med.* **136**, 331.

(These three papers explain the need for macrophages in various aspects of the immune response.)

12

DEVELOPMENT OF B-CELL FUNCTION

OVERVIEW

Up to this point we have examined some of the complexities of the interacting cells in the immune response. In this short chapter we will look at the development of B-cell function. Since antigen selects preprogrammed cells, it is important to know at what stage in the life of the animal that program becomes expressed. To answer this question, analysis of the numbers of precursor cells and the different kinds of clones of effector cells which are generated is important. This chapter will deal with some of the available data on how the immune response begins.

APPEARANCE OF B- AND T-CELLS IN THE NEWBORN

Ig-positive cells first appear in the fetal liver of the mouse by day 17 of gestation. The embryonic thymus has lymphocytes by day 12 of gestation. By day 15 there are both Ig-positive and θ-positive cells in the embryonic spleen. Cells able to bind antigen are found in the embryonic spleen at this time as well. However, the spleens of fetal and newborn mice are not able to generate antibody-producing cells when cultured *in vitro*. This raises the question of whether there are functional precursors present at birth or whether something is preventing them from functioning.

159

DEVELOPMENT OF B-CELL CLONES

In Vitro Spleen Focus Assay

To determine if there are functional *precursors* of antibody-forming cells present in the fetal and newborn mouse, a modification of the focus-forming assay has been carried out *in vitro*. These experiments, presented below, show clearly that the fetal and newborn animal has functional precursors of antibody-forming cells.

In Chapter 10 we discussed the *in vivo* focus-forming assay which showed that there was approximately one antibody-forming precursor cell per 10^6 spleen cells for the antigen SRBC. It has probably not escaped the careful reader that the number of fragments producing antibody and therefore the apparent number of precursors which this method reveals can be limited either by the number of precursors themselves or by the number of helper cells present. Furthermore, the *in vivo* method limits the kinds of analysis which can be carried out on the clones which are generated. A method which overcomes the limitations has been developed by Norman Klinman and his co-workers. This method, the *in vitro* spleen focus assay, is diagrammed in Figure 1.

Mice are carrier primed to generate optimal numbers of helper cells, and these mice are then X-irradiated. It will be recalled from the experiments in Chapter 9 that this method of generating helper cells was used in studying the need for H-2 compatability of B-cells and T-cells. It takes advantage of the fact that carrier-primed helper T-cells are able to carry out helper function after being irradiated if they have been allowed to react with antigen before irradiation. In the present method the carrier-primed, X-irradiated animals are then repopulated with known numbers of adult or neonatal cells to determine the number of precursors of antibody-forming cells present in these cells. This is done by allowing the injected cells to lodge in the spleen of the recipients and 16 hr later removing the spleen and cutting it into small fragments in a manner similar to the *in vivo* focus-forming assay. The method differs from the *in vivo* system because each fragment is then cultured *in vitro* in the presence of hapten conjugated to carrier. The fragments are incubated, and the precursors are allowed to develop into effector cells. The supernatant fluid over each fragment is then assayed for anti-hapten antibody. In this way the number of cells which are able to generate clones of antibody-forming cells are quantitated, and this, by definition, is the number of precursor cells. Because there is an excess of helper cells, each fragment which produces antibody represents a clone of cells making anti-hapten antibody since each clone was derived from a single precursor cell.

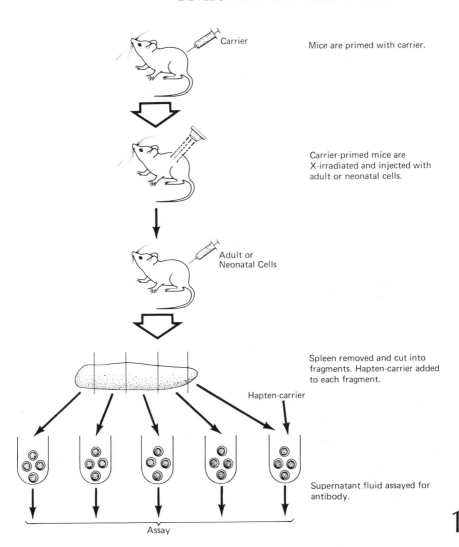

Mice are primed with carrier.

Carrier-primed mice are X-irradiated and injected with adult or neonatal cells.

Adult or Neonatal Cells

Spleen removed and cut into fragments. Hapten-carrier added to each fragment.

Hapten-carrier

Supernatant fluid assayed for antibody.

Assay

In vitro **focus-forming assay.**

Frequency of Precursors in Adults and Newborn

When the *in vitro* focus-forming assay was used to determine the number of precursors to antibody-forming cells to a variety of haptens in adult spleens, it was found that after correcting for cloning efficiency there are approximately 2 to 5 precursors per 10^5 spleen cells. This number is in close agreement with the *in vivo* method. When the number of precursors for haptens was determined for newborn animals, it was found that there is no significant difference in the number of precursors between newborn and adult spleen for some haptens such as DNP and TNP, but at least one other hapten (fluorecine) had 5 to 6 times fewer precursor cells in the neonate. This probably indicates that precursors to different antigens develop at different times.

Clonotypes of Precursor Cells

Antibody molecules of the same specificity can be distinguished from each other by the method of *isoelectric focusing.* In this method the molecules are separated by electrophoresis in a sucrose density gradient which is also a pH gradient. The principle is that the molecules migrate through the pH gradient until they reach the pH at which they have no net charge. They are then collected and analyzed. The pH at which a molecule's charge is neutralized is called the ISOELECTRIC POINT, or pI. Since all the antibody produced by the cells in a fragment are made by cells of the same clone, all these molecules have the same pI. The pI of the antibody molecules produced by the cells which derive from the precursors in the fragments from adult, newborn, and fetal tissue were compared to determine if there was heterogeneity among the clones produced. If two clones produce antibody of different pI but the same antigen-binding specificity, this shows heterogeneity between clones. Each clone producing antibody of the same antigen-binding specificity but of a different pI is termed a CLONOTYPE. All the precursors of anti-DNP give rise to effector cells which produce antibody that specifically binds DNP, but some precursors give rise to progeny producing anti-DNP of different pI values. Since all the antibody produced by a clone is the same, the differences in pI must mean that there are different clones producing anti-DNP antibody.

Klinman and his colleagues have found that before birth and in the neonatal animal there are a limited number of clonotypes for anti-DNP antibody. The number of clonotypes rises the first week after birth. The reason for the increase in clonotypes is not known but could be somatic variation among anti-DNP producing cells (see Chapter 16).

DEVELOPMENT OF ABILITY TO GENERATE ANTIBODY RESPONSES

Immunoincompetence of the Newborn

From the data above it is clear that the newborn spleen has Ig-positive, antigen-binding cells, and θ-positive cells. However, the

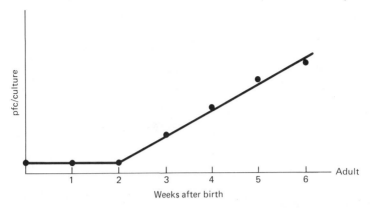

In vitro **anti-SRBC response of spleen cells of different ages. [From Fidler, Chiscon, and Golub (1972).** *J. Immunol.* **109, 136.]**

fact that newborns have impaired immune function has been known for a very long time. For example, spleen cells of newborns are not able to generate antibody responses *in vitro*. As seen in Figure 2, when the *in vitro* anti-SRBC responses of spleen cells of mice of varying ages were compared with adult responses, it was found that not until the mice were over a week of age were they able to generate any antibody response at all and after that time the responses generated were small compared with the responses of adults. It was not until 3 weeks that adult level responses were obtained. Clearly, some form of maturational event is occurring in these spleen cells during the first weeks of life.

Functions of Newborn Macrophages
    To determine if newborn macrophages can function as accessory cells (Chapter 11), an experiment was performed in which adherent cells from the spleens of adult mice were cultured with nonadherent cells from the spleens of newborns. Similarly, adherent cells of newborns were cultured with nonadherent cells of adults. In this manner the ability of the newborn macrophage (adherent cells) to function in antibody formation was determined. This experiment is diagrammed in Figure 3. The results of this study showed that newborn macrophages were equal to adult macrophages in accessory cell function.

Class of Ig on Newborn B-Cells
    The classes of immunoglobulin molecules will be discussed in detail in Chapters 13, 14, and 15. At this point it is important to

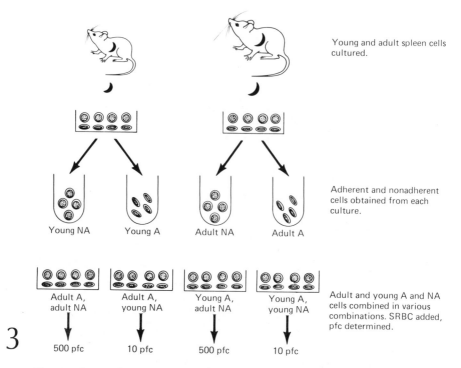

Young and adult spleen cells cultured.

Adherent and nonadherent cells obtained from each culture.

Young NA   Young A   Adult NA   Adult A

Adult A,   Adult A,   Young A,   Young A,
adult NA   young NA   adult NA   young NA

3

500 pfc   10 pfc   500 pfc   10 pfc

Adult and young A and NA cells combined in various combinations. SRBC added, pfc determined.

Comparison of young and adult adherent and nonadherent cells. [After Fidler, Chiscon, and Golub (1972). *J. Immunol.* **109,** 136.]

know that Ig molecules can be distinguished from each other on the basis of *antigenic* differences on one of their peptide chains. Two of these classes, IgM and IgD, appear on the surfaces of B-cells and have been studied on the B-cells of newborn and developing animals. As seen in Figure 4, the spleen B-cells of newborn mice have only IgM molecules. But within a week after birth the number of B-cells with IgD on their surface begins to rise. By 1 month after birth the number of B-cells with IgD is equal to those with IgM. There is also a large group which has *both* IgM and IgD on their surface.

It has been suggested by Vitetta and Uhr that this change in surface Ig class, which is seen to occur during a time of acquisition of function, may be of great developmental significance both in the development of functional B-cells and for the induction of immune tolerance (Chapter 20).

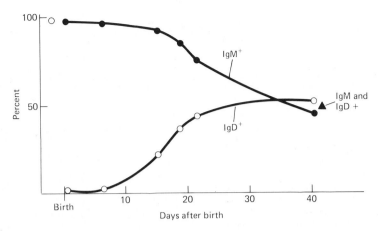

Percentages of IgM-, IgD-positive B-cells in spleens of mice after birth. [From Vitetta *et al.* (1975). *J. Exp. Med.* 141, 206.]

Suppressor Cells in Newborn Spleen

The most probable reason that the young spleen does not produce antibody to thymus-dependent antigens is the presence of *suppressor* T-cells. This class of T-cells is covered in detail in Chapter 18.

SUMMARY

1. B-cells appear in the embryonic fetal liver by day 17 of gestation and in the fetal spleen by day 15. The fetal thymus is lymphoid by day 12, and θ-positive cells are found in the fetal spleen by day 15.
2. By use of an *in vitro* modification of the focus-forming assay, it has been possible to show that newborn and adult animals have comparable numbers of precursors of antibody-forming cells.
3. There are limited numbers of clonotypes before birth, but the diversity of clonotypes increases by a week after birth.
4. Newborn spleens are not able to generate antibody responses even though they have B-cells, T-cells, and macrophages. This is probably due to the presence of suppressor T-cells in the newborn spleen.

READINGS

BOOK

Solomon, J. B. (1971). *Foetal and Neonatal Immunology*, Amsterdam, North-Holland Publishing Co.

ARTICLES

Press, J. L., and Klinman, N. R. (1974). Frequency of hapten-specific B-cells in neonatal and adult murine spleens, *Eur. J. Immunol.* **4,** 155. (The enumeration of B-cell precursors by an *in vitro* method.)

Klinman, N. R., and Press, J. L. (1975). The characterization of the B-cell repertoire specific for the 2,4-dinitrophenyl and 2,4,6-trinitrophenyl determinants in neonatal BALB/c mice, *J. Exp. Med.* **141,** 1133. (Analysis of clonotypes of the B-cell precursor population.)

Fidler, J. M., Chiscon, M. O., and Golub, E. S. (1972). Functional development of the interacting cells in the immune response. II. Development of immunocompetence to heterologous erythrocytes *in vitro, J. Immunol.* **109,** 136. (Development of the immune response.)

Vitetta, E. S., Melcher, U., McWilliams, M., Lamm, M. E., Phillips-Quagliata, J. M., and Uhr, J. W. (1975). Cell surface immunoglobulin. XI. The appearance of an IgD-like molecule on murine lymphoid cells during ontogeny, *J. Exp. Med.* **141,** 206. (The possible developmental role of IgD on cell surfaces.)

Spear, P. G., Wang, A., Ruitshauer, U., and Edelman, G. M. (1973). Characterization of splenic lymphoid cells in fetal and newborn mice, *J. Exp. Med.* **138,** 557.

III

IMMUNOGLOBULINS

Textbooks of immunology traditionally start with material on the structure of immunoglobulin (Ig) molecules. Because the emphasis in this book is on the cellular basis of the immune response, cell cooperation was stressed at the outset. However, the student of immunology must be familiar with the product of the B-cell, the antibody molecule, because understanding a good deal of the cellular basis of cooperation and control depends on knowledge of the structure of the immunoglobulin molecule. Furthermore, it was evident in Chapter 10 that the T-cell receptor may be part of an Ig molecule. The next few years will undoubtedly see a great deal of immunochemistry being carried out on these membrane-associated Ig molecules.

Immunoglobulins are the class of proteins which contain antibody activity. The basic immunoglobulin molecule is a four-chain structure held together by disulfide bonds. There are two heavy chains (H chains) and two light chains (L chains). The molecular weights of Ig molecules range from 160,000 to 1,000,000. The classes of Ig are defined, however, not by their molecular weight but by antigenic differences in their H chains. There are five classes of Ig molecules: IgG, IgM, IgA, IgD, and IgE. All have antibody activity, but they vary in the other functions which Ig molecules carry out such as fixation to tissues.

When the amino acid sequences of individual Ig molecules are compared, it is found that the molecules of one class of Ig have large areas of common sequence. These areas are called the constant

167

regions (C regions). However, there is a small area of the molecules in which the sequence of amino acids varies among different Ig molecules. This area is called the variable region (V region). Antigen binding is in the V region. Within V regions there are areas of constancy and areas of hypervariability. The hypervariability regions provide the structural basis of antibody specificity.

The great unanswered question is how the diversity of areas which code for antibody specificity are generated. One theory, the germ-line theory, states that genes for all specificities are passed from generation to generation in the germ cells (sperm and egg). Another says that only a few genes for antibody are passed via sperm and egg and that diversity is generated in somatic cells.

13

STRUCTURE OF IMMUNOGLOBULINS

OVERVIEW

The product of the B-cell is the antibody molecule. These molecules are found in the globulin fraction of serum and are called immunoglobulins (Ig). In this chapter we will see that monomeric forms of Ig molecules have a characteristic four-chain structure. The antigen-combining region is at one end of the molecule, and the ability to combine with complement as well as carry out other biological functions is at the other end. Ig molecules are heterogeneous. Their antigenic heterogeneity provides a means of categorizing them on the basis of class. All members of the species have all classes of Ig. There is further heterogeneity which is genetically controlled within the species called allotypic variation. Further heterogeneity is found in idiotypic variation, which defines Ig molecules on the basis of the unique antigenic character of their combining region. This chapter will cover some details of the structure and heterogeneity of immunoglobulin molecules.

ANTIBODIES AND IMMUNOGLOBULINS

Serum, the fluid portion of blood, can be fractionated by a variety of means into its several protein components. The major proteins of the serum are albumin and globulins. The globulin fraction can be subfractionated by electrophoresis on the basis of charge into α-, β-, and γ-globulins. *Antibodies* are found primarily in the γ-globulins.

169

This fact was shown very elegantly in 1939 by Tselius and Kabat. The electrophoretic pattern of the serum from rabbits which had been immunized to antigen was determined before the antiserum was reacted with antigen. The antigen was then added, the precipitated antigen-antibody complex was removed, and the electrophoretic pattern again determined. By observing which protein components were removed from the serum by binding with antigen, it was possible to determine which fraction contained the antibody molecules. As seen in Figure 1, the gamma globulin fraction was selectively reduced after reaction with antigen. This indicated that antibodies were found in the gamma globulin fraction. Since all gamma globulins may be antibodies to some antigen, it was decided to call this heterogeneous group of molecules IMMUNOGLOBULINS.

CHAIN STRUCTURE OF IMMUNOGLOBULINS

Cleavage with Proteolytic Enzymes

The immunoglobulin molecule (commonly referred to as Ig) is one of the most extensively studied of all the large protein molecules. The approach which has been so successful in determining the structure of the Ig molecule (and which has led to the Nobel prize for two of the prime movers in the field) has been to split the molecule chemically and then to separate and analyze the products. One of these Nobel prize winners, R. R. Porter in England, treated rabbit antibody with the proteolytic enzyme *papain* and separated the products on the basis of their charge on a carboxymethylcellulose column. Three fragments, called I, II, and III, were obtained. Molecular weight determination by ultracentrifugation showed the undigested Ig to have a molecular weight of 188,000. Fragments I and II had molecular weights of approximately 50,000, and fragment III had a molecular weight of 80,000. Fragments I and II were able to bind specifically with antigen and were called *Fab* (fragment with antigen binding). Fragment III did not react with antigen but did react with complement and was crystallizable. This fragment was called *Fc* (fragment which can be crystallized). It was known from immunological antiquity (pre-1960) that most antibody is bivalent, i.e., has two antigen-binding sites, and that after reaction with antigen it can bind or fix complement. Porter and his co-workers therefore proposed a model for the antibody molecule built on the papain fragmentation studies which gave a structural basis for both antigen binding and complement fixation. This model is seen in Figure 2.

Treatment of the antibody molecule with another proteolytic enzyme, *pepsin,* gave different cleavage products. In studies by Nisonoff

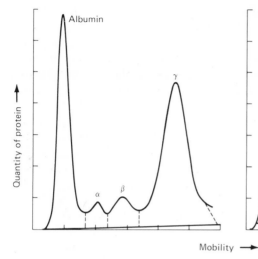
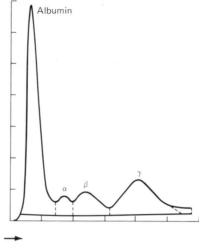

Electrophoretic analysis of rabbit anti-egg albumin antiserum before and after reaction of the antiserum with the antigen. Note that the gamma globulin fraction is selectively reduced after reaction with antigen. [From Tiselius and Kabat (1939). *J. Exp. Med.* **69,** 119.]

and his colleagues the 7s antibody molecule was only slightly lowered in molecular weight after treatment with pepsin. One 5s fragment and many small peptides were obtained. The 5s fragment retained all the antigen-binding capacity of the original molecule. When the 5s fragment was treated with agents that reduce disulfide bonds, the 5s fragment was split into two fragments of equal size, each of which reacted with antigen. It seemed probable from these studies that

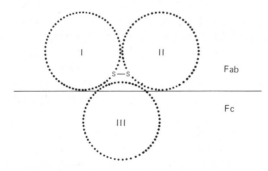

2

Initial diagrammatic representation of the structure of the immunoglobulin molecule obtained from papain cleavage studies.

these fragments were equivalent to fragments I and II of the papain treatment, and this suggested that fragments I and II were joined by disulfide bonds. The importance of the disulfide bonds in the molecule is seen from papain digestion experiments using a different form of papain than that used in the original studies. In the original studies of Porter the papain was activated (as all papain must be) with thiol before it was used, and the thiol was present throughout the cleavage process. When the papain studies were carried out with insoluble papain where it was possible to wash away the unreacted thiol after the papain was activated, there was little cleavage of the molecule. However, if thiol was added to the insoluble papain-treated antibody preparation after the insoluble papain had been removed, the molecule was split into three fragments. This shows that the proteolytic enzyme had cleaved parts of the molecule but that they were still held together by disulfide bonds. Only in the presence of an agent which reduced these disulfide bonds was it possible to see separation of the fragments.

Reduction and Alkylation Studies

The other Nobel prize winner for work on immunoglobulin structure, G. M. Edelman of the Rockefeller University, showed the importance of the disulfide bonds in studies in which the immunoglobulin molecule was allowed to unfold in 6 *M urea*. The disulfide bonds were then reduced with mercaptoethanol. The reduced molecule was treated with an alkylating agent to prevent the disulfide bonds from reforming, and the reduced and alkylated chains of the molecule were then studied by a variety of physical, chemical, and immunochemical techniques. These reduction and alkylation studies allowed the chains of the molecule to be dissociated from each other and separated on Sephadex columns or by gel electrophoresis. Edelman and his co-workers quickly found that there were two components to the immunoglobulin molecule. One component had a molecular weight of approximately 20,000 and the other of approximately 50,000. The heavy component was called the *H*, or *heavy chain* and the lighter was called *L*, or *light chain*. The relative concentrations of H and L chains and the molecular weight of the intact molecule were consistent with a molecule which has *four chains,* two H and two L.

Relationship between Fab, Fc, H, and L

By producing antibodies against whole gamma globulin, Fab, and Fc, it was possible to determine the relationship between the H and L chains obtained by reduction and alkylation and the fragments obtained by papain digestion. The L chain reacted with anti-Fab antiserum but not with anti-Fc. The H chain, however, reacted with both anti-Fab and anti-Fc. This shows that the H chain is shared by Fab and Fc but the L chain is unique to Fab. The model which emerged by incorporating these observations is seen in Figure 3. The chains are connected by interchain disulfide bridges.

The number and exact position of the *inter-heavy chain* disulfide bridges, i.e., the disulfide bonds holding the H chain together, may vary between different immunoglobulin molecules. They are usually in a region near the middle of the heavy chain which is unusually high in proline content. This area is called the HINGE REGION because this area, which is close to the site of susceptibility to proteolytic enzymes, is thought to be a flexible portion of the molecule.

Figure 4 is a more extensive diagrammatic model of the immunoglobulin molecule with each of the parts labeled. Note that the area of the heavy chain in the Fab portion of the molecule is called the *Fd* region.

All vertebrate species which have immunoglobulins have a similar immunoglobulin structure. The most primitive species that has been well studied is an elasmobranch, the smooth dogfish *(Mastelus canis)*. The immunoglobulin molecule of this species is composed of four chains, two light and two heavy, as are the immunoglobulins of the higher forms. The question of the evolution of the immunoglobulin molecule will be discussed in Chapter 15.

CLASSES OF IMMUNOGLOBULINS

Heterogeneity of Ig Molecules

Antibody activity is found in a broad spectrum of immunoglobulins. When analyzed by *ultracentrifugation,* antibody activity is found in molecules with sedimentation coefficients ranging from 7s to 19s.

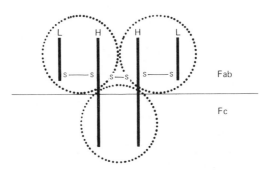

3

A model of the immunoglobulin molecule incorporating the proteolytic digestion studies and the reduction and alkylation studies. The model shows the relationship between Fab, Fc, H, and L.

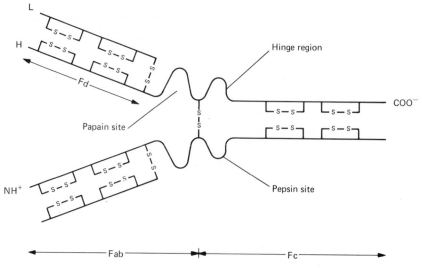

Diagrammatic presentation of the Ig molecule.

These correspond to molecular weights ranging from approximately 150,000 to over 1,000,000. By zone *electrophoresis* great heterogeneity is observed in these molecules, indicating a heterogeneity in charge. When immunoglobulins of one species are injected into an animal of another species, they act as antigens. The antibody which is raised against globulins can be used as reagent to study the antigenic heterogeneity of the globulin molecules. This antigenic hetero-geneity has proven to be a most useful means of studying the immunoglobulins.

Definition of Class

The immunoglobulins are classified according to their antigenic properties. Antibodies against the immunoglobulins of one species, man, for example, can be raised in a rabbit. Since, as we already stated, there is great heterogeneity among immunoglobulin mole-cules, such an antiserum will contain antibodies against all the classes of immunoglobulin in the serum. The different reactivities are visualized by gel diffusion precipitation reaction. Immunoelec-trophoresis is the most common method. In this technique presence of antigens is demonstrated by means of precipitation zones with anti-body. In a typical pattern there are several bands of precipitate, each representing a *class* of immunoglobulin. All normal individuals bear molecules of each class in their serum.

Use of Myeloma Proteins

The fact that normal serum contains representatives of each of the immunoglobulin classes makes it difficult to produce antisera which react with only one class of immunoglobulin. The use of *myeloma proteins* has helped overcome this difficulty. Multiple myeloma is a disease in which there is a very high concentration of only one class of immunoglobulin (the myeloma protein) in the patient's serum. The molecules are of only one class and are physically and chemically homogeneous. Because of this homogeneity it is inferred that the cells producing the immunoglobulins are derived from a single clone; i.e., they are all descended from a single cell. This unfortunate "experiment of nature" gives us access to high concentrations of immunoglobulin molecules of the same class. By producing antibodies against myeloma proteins (immunoglobulins), it has been possible to develop reagent antisera and also to identify classes of immunoglobulins which are present in very low concentration in normal serum.

Classes

As noted above the class of an immunoglobulin is determined by its unique antigenic properties. The antigens which define class are located on the heavy chain of the immunoglobulin molecule. There are five classes of immunoglobulins, and they are designated by capital Roman letters: IgG, IgM, IgA, IgD, and IgE (Ig, of course, stands for immunoglobulin). The H chain of each class is designated by the small Greek letter corresponding to the Roman letter of the class. Thus, the H chain of IgG is a γ chain, the H chain of IgM is a μ chain, IgA has an α chain, IgD has a δ chain, and IgE has an ϵ chain.

We will see below that many of the classes are polymers of the basic four-chain structure described in the previous section and have different molecular weights and other biological properties. None of these other qualities define class. The class of an immunoglobulin is always determined by its H-chain antigens.

The light chains of immunoglobulin molecules have two antigenic varieties. These are called κ and λ. All classes of immunoglobulin have these two types of L chains. Each monomeric immunoglobulin molecule has two L chains which are linked to the H chains by disulfide bonds. A given immunoglobulin molecule has two of the same type of L chains, either κ or λ, and never contains one κ chain and one λ chain. The monomeric form of any immunoglobulin molecule can therefore be described by its chain structure. An IgG molecule, for example, will always have two γ chains and may have two κ chains or two λ chains. It would thus be $\gamma 2\kappa 2$ or $\gamma 2\lambda 2$.

We said earlier that the molecular weights of the immunoglobulins varied from 150,000 to 1,000,000. This variation in molecular weight is due to *polymerization* of the basic monomeric unit which we have been describing. An IgM molecule, for example, has a molecular weight of approximately 1,000,000. IgM is a pentamer of the basic monomer structure (but it must be emphasized, not five IgG monomers polymerized). Since the monomer of IgM is $\mu 2\kappa 2$ or $\mu 2\lambda 2$, IgM is described as $(\mu 2\kappa 2)5$ or $(\mu 2\lambda 2)5$. IgA may have a variable number of monomeric units polymerized into a large molecule and would be designated as $(\alpha 2\kappa 2)n$ or $(\alpha 2\lambda 2)n$, where n can range from 2 to 5.

Subclasses

Antisera have been obtained which distinguish between molecules within a class. We saw above that the proper reagent antiserum can identify Ig molecules which have γ chains and therefore belong to IgG class. However, when these IgG molecules are reacted with antisera which have been produced to detect differences *within* the class, it is possible to detect differences among γ chains. These differences define *subclasses* of H chains and thus subclasses of immunoglobulins. Two molecules may be IgG, that is, each contains two γ chains, but the chains of the two IgG molecules may differ from each other antigenically as well as in biological properties. In man, for example, there are four known γ-chain subclasses called IgG1, IgG2, IgG3, and IgG4. Every normal individual has all subclasses of immunoglobulin in his serum.

In the guinea pig there are two types of γ chains, $\gamma 1$ and $\gamma 2$, which were first identified by immunoelectrophoresis. These two subclasses of IgG have different biological properties. While both will bind antigen, it can be shown that $\gamma 1$ will fix to skin and sensitize an animal for local antigen-antibody reactions, called passive cutaneous anaphylaxis reactions, but will not bind complement or be able to elicit another kind of allergic skin reaction called an Arthus reaction. Guinea pig $\gamma 2$, however, is able to bind complement and can induce an Arthus reaction but will not sensitize an animal for a passive cutaneous anaphylaxis reaction.

In all cases where subclasses of immunoglobulin molecules have been found, the antigenic differences have been located on the H chain, either in the Fc or the Fd portion.

ALLOTYPIC AND IDIOTYPIC VARIATION

Allotypes

Allotypes are genetically controlled antigenic determinants on immunoglobulin molecules. An allotype is a series of antigens coded for at one genetic locus. The entire series of antigens is expressed within a species, but one individual will express only a few of the antigens coded at that locus. Most species have allotypic determinants. Family studies have shown that these antigenic determinants on immunoglobulins are inherited in a Mendelian fashion. The fact that they are inherited as autosomal, allelic characters led to the name *allotype*, although the word has not been found much in the genetic literature. These genetically controlled differences have proved to be a useful tool in understanding the genetic control of immunoglobulin synthesis.

In man there are two major allotypic groups, *Gm* and *InV*, and one minor group which is closely associated with Gm, called *Am*. InV is found on the light chain and thus occurs on IgG, IgM, and IgA. Gm, on the other hand, is associated with heavy chains and appears only on γ chains. This allotype is therefore limited to IgG molecules. There are approximately 25 Gm specificities, and they have unique distributions on subclasses of IgG. For example, Gm(a), (x), (f), and (z) occur only on IgG1. These markers are of great value in mapping the genes controlling the synthesis of the H and L chains.

A single amino acid difference distinguishes InV(1) from InV(3). In the Gm system heavy chains from IgG1 individuals who are Gm(a)+ have a peptide which IgG1 heavy chains from Gm(a)− individuals lack. When compared with H chains from IgG2 and IgG3 individuals who always lack Gm(a), it is found that a Gm "non-a" peptide is associated with these chains, whereas a Gm "a" peptide is associated with Gm(a)+ chains. Amino acid analysis of the Gm "a" peptide and the Gm "non-a" peptide indicates a difference of two amino acids.

In rabbits there appear to be about eight gene loci for allotypic determinants. The specificity associated with the *a* locus is found in all classes of immunoglobulins in the variable region of the heavy chain (see below). Specificities associated with the *d* locus are found in the constant region of Fd, and those with the *e* locus on the Fc portion of the γ chain. The b specificities are found on κ chains, and the c specificities on the λ chains of all classes. Specificities associated with f are found on IgA. Immunoglobulin molecules of IgG, IgM, and IgA all share the b specificity as would be expected from their position on the L chain. The *a* group specificity, which is associated with H chains, is shared by the γ, μ, and α chains (unlike the Gm specificity in man). This sharing of the *a* allotype by several H chains is known as the TODD PHENOMENON.

There are four known allotype loci in the mouse. The markers are all located on the constant region of the H chain. Markers on IgG$_{2a}$,

IgG$_{2b}$, IgG$_1$, and IgA have been identified, but none have been found for the H chain of IgM or for mouse L chains. Mouse allotypes have been especially useful because congenic mice, which differ only at the allotype locus, can be used in cell transfer experiments where cells are transferred across histocompatability barriers.

Idiotypes

So far in this chapter we have seen that there are antigenic determinants on the H chain which are unique to each class of immunoglobulins. Each normal member of a species has all the immunoglogulin classes in its serum. Some members of the species have antigenic determinants on their immunoglobulin which other members do not. These are the allotypic determinants. There is yet another kind of antigenic determinant on immunoglobulin molecules which is unique to particular molecules of an individual. Called IDIOTYPIC DETERMINANTS, each is determined by a unique amino acid sequence. The unique sequence of amino acids is found in the antigen-combining site of the antibody molecule. Like class and allotypic determinants, idiotypic determinants are identified by the ability to raise an antibody against them. For example, an animal is

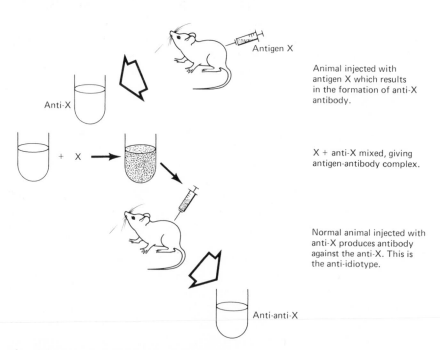

Animal injected with antigen X which results in the formation of anti-X antibody.

X + anti-X mixed, giving antigen-antibody complex.

Normal animal injected with anti-X produces antibody against the anti-X. This is the anti-idiotype.

5

Production of anti-idiotype antibody.

injected with an antigen and the antibody collected. This antibody is then reacted *in vitro* with the antigen, thus forming antigen-antibody complexes, which are then injected into another animal. This animal produces antibody against the antigen in the antigen-antibody complex, but, more important for our purpose, it also produces antibody against a small segment of the *antibody* part of the complex. Since both animals are of the same species, each contains all the classes of immunoglobulin and will therefore not make any anti-class specific antibody. If they are of the same allotypes, they will not produce any anti-allotype antibody. The antibody produced by the animal immunized with the antigen-antibody complex must therefore be directed against a unique portion of the antibody molecule. This unique portion is the antigen-combining site of the antibody molecule.

The anti-idiotype antibody raised in this way will not react with any other immunoglobulins in the donor other than those which have antibody activity against the antigen used; thus we see that it is unique to those immunoglobulins which have specific antibody activity. This is diagrammed in Figure 5.

SUMMARY

1. Antibodies are found in the globulin fraction of serum. The globulin molecules of serum are called immunoglobulins (Ig).
2. The monomeric form of the Ig molecule is a four-chain structure. There are two heavy chains (H chains) and two light chains (L chains). The chains are held together by disulfide bonds.
3. There is great physical, chemical, and antigenic heterogeneity among Ig molecules. The class of Ig is determined by antigenic differences.
4. There are five classes of Ig called IgG, IgM, IgA, IgD, and IgE. Normal individuals have each of the classes present in their serum.
5. Homogeneous populations of Ig classes are obtained through the use of myeloma proteins.
6. Allotypes are a series of antigens found on Ig molecules which are coded for at one genetic locus. Each member of a species expresses only a few of the antigens.
7. Idiotypes are unique sequences on Ig molecules and are found in the antigen-combining site.

READINGS

REVIEWS

Porter, R. R. (1973). Structural studies of immunoglobulins, *Science,* **180,** 713.

Edelman, G. M. (1973). Antibody structure and molecular immunology, *Science,* **180,** 830.

(Nobel prize lectures of two of the prime movers of the field.)

Kochwa, S., and Kunkel, H. G. (1971). Immunoglobulins, *Ann. N.Y. Acad. Sci.,* Vol. 190. (Series of papers on all aspects of structure of immunoglobulins.)

Natvig, J. B., and Kunkel, H. G. (1973). Human immunoglobulins: Classes, subclasses, genetic variants, and idiotypes, *Adv. Immunol.* **16,** 1. (A review of class and allotype.)

Hopper, J. E., and Nisonoff, A. (1971). Individual antigenic specificity of immunoglobulins, *Adv. Immunol.* **13,** 57. (A review of idiotypes.)

Kindt, T. (1975). Rabbit immunoglobulin allotypes: Structure, immunology, and genetics, *Adv. Immunol.* **21,** 35.

14

STRUCTURAL BASIS OF ANTIBODY
SPECIFICITY

OVERVIEW

So far in this section we have discussed the chain structure and antigenic composition of Ig molecules. Obviously, the main concern of the study of the structure of antibody molecule is to understand the structural basis of specific combination with antigen. The H and L chains of Ig molecules can be divided into variable and constant regions. The variable regions provide an enormous range of amino acid sequences and hence antigen-combining sites. In this chapter we will discuss the means by which this problem has been attacked and solved.

SEQUENCE STUDIES OF IMMUNOGLOBULINS

Primary Structure

It is known from studies in protein chemistry that the secondary and tertiary structures of polypeptides are determined by the primary structure. *Primary structure* is the sequence of amino acids in the peptide chain. *Secondary* and *tertiary* structure are the folding of the chain and the shape of the molecule. We also know from studies in molecular biology that the primary structure of a peptide chain is a direct reflection of the nucleic acid base sequences in the DNA which codes for the peptide. Because of this, a detailed understanding of the primary sequence of immunoglobulin molecules is essential to understand the nature of the combining site for antigen as well as the organization of the DNA which codes for the sites.

181

Since the serum of a normal individual contains all the classes of Ig, there is great heterogeneity (class, subclass, allotype, and idiotype). This makes the study of the amino acid sequence of serum immunoglobulin molecules very difficult. The use of myeloma proteins which are homogeneous has allowed the problem to be overcome, and the complete amino acid sequence of many light chains and a few entire molecules are known. BENCE JONES PROTEINS, which are light chains excreted in the urine of certain patients with multiple myeloma, have provided the material from which much of the sequence data on immunoglobulin molecules has come. A point of departure for studies of the structural basis of antibody specificity is the fact that myeloma proteins and Bence Jones proteins are really normal products of abnormal cells. Because of this one can study the product of these cells' normal immunoglobulins but with none of the heterogeneity found in immunoglobulins obtained from normal serum.

Constant and Variable Regions

Since antibodies combine specifically with antigen and an animal can make antibodies to an enormous number of antigens, there must be some structural basis for this property. One of the discoveries crucial to solving this problem was the finding that there are regions of constancy and variability in amino acid sequence of the immunoglobulin molecule. The announcement of the discovery was one of those rare moments in science when everyone is aware of an important advance. Russel Doolittle describes the moment:

Early in 1965 a meeting of the Antibody Workshop was held at Warner Springs, California, a small resort community about 60 miles east of San Diego. The meeting, with about 80 persons in attendance, was unique on several counts. Largely organized by Melvin Cohn (of the Salk Institute), a determined effort had been made to infiltrate the immunologic ranks with a galaxy of stellar molecular biologists, including James Watson, Francis Crick, Christian Anfinsen, Max Delbrück, Seymour Benzer, and a dozen other nonimmunologists of high repute. The program was simple enough—a few talks on immunologically competent cells, immunogenetics, antibody structure, and the like. For the first two days everything went according to schedule, predictable progress—but not much more—being reported, and the sessions were only slightly lengthened by the presence of the imported Brain Trust. On the third morning, however, the assemblage was electrified by the unexpected announcement from Norbert Hilschmann, reporting on work he had done in Lyman Craig's laboratory, that he had virtually completed the amino acid sequences of two very different Bence Jones proteins (the equivalent of antibody light chains), and, with one quite explicable exception, had found that all the many amino acid replacements had occurred in the amino-terminal half of the molecules. Clearly, immunoglobulin light chains had a variable half and a constant half.

The impact on the meeting was instantaneous, something very close to pandemonium ensuing. Francis Crick made his way to the chalkboard and drew a flurry of twisted loops, implying that simple DNA rearrangements could now explain antibody diversity; Seymour Benzer declared that at last immunology had become a science. It was one of those rare moments when an entire group senses that a solution to a major problem is directly at hand but no one is quite sure of how to put the last piece in the puzzle, or even how to find it. Surely if only a few more sequences were obtained the pattern would become absolutely clear. [R. Doolittle (1974). *Science,* **183,** 190, review of Smith, The Variation and Adaptive Expression of Antibodies.]

In other words, when the first amino acid from the amino terminal end of Bence Jones protein A and protein B are compared, there is a different amino acid at this position in each of the proteins. Similarly, when the second, third, etc., positions are compared, the amino acids at each of these positions are different in each protein. This difference at each position continues until roughly the midpoint of the light chain. From that point on there is complete correspondence of amino acids, position for position, except for the genetically controlled allotypic variations already mentioned. Thus the first amino acid beyond the midpoint in proteins A and B are identical. This correspondence holds until the carboxy terminal end of the chain. The light chain could therefore be divided into a *variable* half and a *constant* half (variable and constant in terms of comparing the amino acid sequence of one Bence Jones protein to the amino acid sequence of another Bence Jones protein). The variable or *V region* starts as the amino terminal end of the chain and comprises the first 100 or so amino acids of the light chain. The constant or *C region* begins at around residue 100 and continues to the carboxy terminal end of the molecule.

The H chain also has a C region and a V region. The V region is at the amino terminal end and extends for the same length as the V regions of the L chain (approximately 100 amino acids). The C region of the H chain is longer than the C region of the L chain. In fact, the C region of the H chain is roughly three times as long as the C region of the L chain or the V region of the H chain.

The chains of the immunoglobulin molecule can thus be divided into their V and C components so that a light chain consists of two parts, V_L and C_L (variable$_{light}$ and constant$_{light}$). Similarly, the heavy chain can be divided into V_H and C_H. An extensive diagram of an Ig monomer is seen in Figure 1.

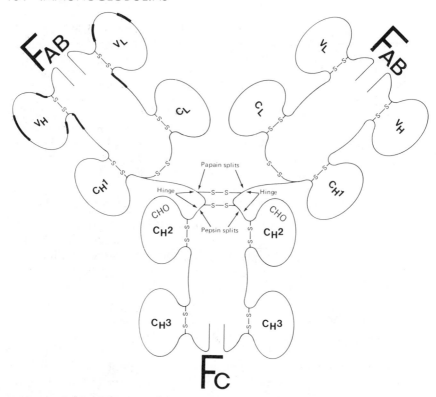

1

A model of the immunoglobulin molecule. From Kabat (1973). 3rd Int. Convoc. Immunol., Buffalo, N.Y., 1972. Karger, Basel.

Homology Studies

The sequence of the C_H region is more complex than the amino acid sequence of the C_L region since the C_H is three times as long as the C_L. By an analysis of the amino acid sequences of the C_H region of a single myeloma protein Edelman and his co-workers showed that the C_H region is approximately 330 amino acids long and is composed of three C_H subregions, each with great *homology* for the other (see below). Thus the C_H can be divided into heavy-chain common regions 1, 2, and 3 (C_H1, C_H2, and C_H3). Each of the regions contains an *intrachain* disulfide bridge spanning 60 amino acids. The length of the individual regions is 110 amino acids. The V_L and V_H regions also contain an intrachain disulfide and are the same length as each of the C_H regions (see Figure 1).

The reason for considering the constant region to be three subregions comes from analysis of the amino acid sequences in each of the parts for *homology*. Homologous sequences of amino acids are those which show more similarity than could occur by chance. By use of a computer analysis which was developed for comparing sequences of different chains of a molecule, the parts of the Ig molecule can be compared to determine if the chains have similarities in sequence composition which are greater than could be expected to occur by chance. When two parts of a chain of the Ig molecule can be compared in this way if they do have such similarities, this could argue for a common ancestral gene for the two sequences. For example, the chains of hemoglobin have different amino acid sequences, but it is known that there once was a single ancestral gene which underwent tandem duplication, giving two peptides of the same amino acid sequence. During evolutionary time each of the two genes underwent different mutations so that the peptides for which the genes code are different at the present time. Knowing the dictionary of nucleic acid base sequences for each amino acid, one can determine the number of mutations needed to go from one amino acid to another. By determining the minimal number of mutations required to change one amino acid to another, it has been possible to draw conclusions about the history of the genes involved in coding for peptides.

In the case of the immunoglobulins, the amino acid sequence of a portion of one part of a chain was compared with the amino acid sequence of a portion of the chain elsewhere in the molecule. This was possible because the complete amino acid sequence of this protein was known. In this manner the amino acid sequence of an area in one part of the C_H was compared with a sequence of amino acids in another part of the C_H region. Similarly, the V_L region was compared with the C_L region or the V_H region, etc. This laborious analysis was carried out by computer until all possible comparisons had been made. The minimal number of mutations required to go from one amino acid to another was determined and plotted against the cumulative frequency of each minimal number of mutations required.

From this analysis three *domains* within the constant region of the H chain were defined. Each of these domains contained an *intrachain disulfide bridge* (in contrast to an *interchain* bridge). These intrachain disulfide bridges cause a loop in the chain. Furthermore, there is sequence homology between the three regions, meaning that even though their amino acid sequences are not identical, the differences between them can be explained by one or two mutational events in the DNA triplet coding for the amino acid. This finding is consistent with the notion that the three C_H regions had a common ancestral gene which through evolutionary time had undergone tandem duplication. Each of the duplicated regions has then undergone independent mutation.

STRUCTURAL BASIS OF ANTIGEN BINDING

Hypervariable Regions

With the realization that the immunoglobulin molecule contained variable regions, it became immediately apparent that this could be the structural basis for antigen binding. If there were total variability at all 100 or so amino acids in the V region, the permutations of possible structures becomes astronomic. It was already known that the antigen binding area was in the Fab and that the V regions are found in the Fab.

As more light chains were sequenced, it became apparent that the variable region was not totally variable. Comparison of sequences between different light chains revealed that there were some invariant areas within the V region. These areas, however, could be grouped into families. A V REGION FAMILY is a group of light chains from individual myelomas having stretches of amino acids in their V regions which are similar or identical. If the amino acid sequence of the V region of a representative light chain from one family is compared with the V region sequence of a member of the same light chain family, there is a great amount of common sequence. When compared with the V region sequence of another light chain family, however, there is little common sequence.

Wu and Kabat in 1970 compared all the then existing sequences of V_L families and found that there are three areas which are always variable. These were called the HYPERVARIABLE REGIONS or "hot spots." It is these hypervariable regions that are the structural basis of antigen binding.

Nature of the Active Site

The study of the nature of the antigen-binding site has been approached in a variety of ways. One of these is by *affinity labeling* of the site, a method developed by Wofsy and Singer. Antigen binds to antibody by noncovalent interaction (H bonding, van der Waals forces, etc.). The principle of affinity labeling is to construct a modified hapten which has the property not only of binding to antibody but, once initial binding has occurred, of forming a *covalent* bond with an amino acid at the site of binding. The covalent bond forms preferentially at the site of closest contact of the modified hapten and the antibody, i.e., the site with the greatest affinity for the hapten. This site, by definition, is the antigen-binding site. By analyzing the structures of the immunoglobulin molecule which have bound the hapten, it was found that both H and L chains make a contribution to the binding of the antigen at the combining site since affinity label can be found covalently linked to both chains.

Size of the Antigen-Combining Site

Some of the earliest attempts to determine the *size* of the combining site were carried out by inhibition of antigen-antibody reactions using logic similar to that in competitive inhibition of enzyme-substrate interactions. In the classic studies of Kabat and his co-workers anti-dextran antibody (a large molecule of repeating sugar subunits) binds to dextran. Smaller subunits of the dextran (3, 4, 5, etc., sugar subunits) were then added to the antibody. If the small molecule could react with the combining site on the antibody molecule when the large dextran molecule was added, the combining site would be filled with the small molecule and the large molecule would be prevented from reacting. By using a graded series of sizes of dextran subunits, it was found that in general the site was fully occupied (inhibition approached maximum) by a molecule of 7 sugar subunits. Similar experiments with other antigen-antibody systems using small subunits of the various antigens showed that the combining site could have dimensions of about 30 Å × 10 Å × 6Å.

Shape of the Antibody Molecule

Historically the antigen-binding site on an antibody molecule has been thought of in terms of a lock and key in which a cavity, the combining site, is filled with the antigenic determinant. This rather simple-minded notion has turned out to be essentially correct. The three-dimensional shape of the Ig molecule and the combining site have been established by X-ray diffraction analysis.

The general three-dimensional view of the Ig molecule which came from the correlation of the sequence, homology, and diffraction studies is seen in Figure 2. Analysis of the electron density maps of the Fab fragment showed that each homology unit (that is, V_H, V_L,

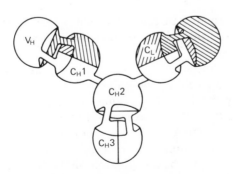

2

Shape of the Ig monomer obtained from X-ray differentiation studies. [From Poliak *et al.* (1972). *Nature, New Biol.* 235, 137.]

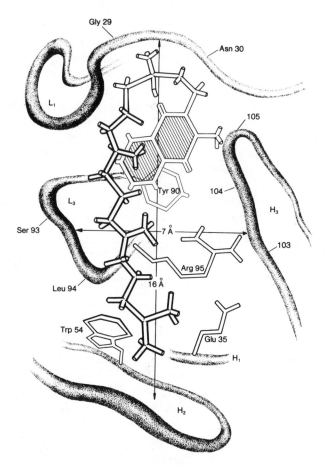

3

Schematic view of the antigen-combining site of an antibody molecule. [From Amzel *et al.* (1974). *P.N.A.S.* 71, 1427.]

C_H, C_L) had a characteristic folding which is termed the IMMUNOGLOBU-LIN FOLD. The structural domains are thus seen to have a common pattern.

In V_L and V_H units the hypervariable regions are found around residues 25, 50, and 100. In the Fab of a human myeloma, which has been extensively studied, the regions around these residues have been shown to form a cleft approximately 20Å × 25 Å. This is not too far from the size estimated for the combining site by competition experiments. The combining site with a hapten (vitamin K) bound to the site is seen in Figure 3. It is possible that one of the hypervariable regions may be the primary binding site and the other two may act as stabilizing sites.

SUMMARY

1. Amino acid sequence studies of Ig chains show that both light and heavy chains have variable and constant regions.
2. Antigen binding is in the hypervariable portions of the variable regions.
3. Both H and L chains participate in antigen binding.

READINGS

BOOK

Kabat, E. A. (1968). *Structural Concepts in Immunology and Immunochemistry,* New York, Holt, Rinehart and Winston. (A masterful summary of the structural basis of specificity.)

REVIEWS

Capra, J. D., and Kehoe, J. M. (1975). Hypervariable regions, idiotypy, and antibody-combining site, *Adv. Immunol.* **20,** 1.

Dorrington, K. J., and Tanford, C. (1970). Molecular and size conformation of immunoglobulins, *Adv. Immunol.* **12,** 333.

Givol, D. (1973). Structural analysis of the antibody combining site, *Contemp. Top. Mol. Immunol.* **2,** 27.

Kehoe, J. M. and Capra, J. D. (1974). Phylogenetic aspects of immunoglobulin variable region diversity, *Contemp. Top. Mol. Immunol.* **3,** 143.

Poljak, R. J. (1975). X-ray diffraction studies of immunoglobulins, *Adv. Immunol.* **21,** 1.

ARTICLE

Wu, T. T. E., and Kabat, E. A. (1970). An analysis of the sequences of the variable regions of Bence Jones proteins and myeloma light chains and their implications for antibody complementarity, *J. Exp. Med.* **132,** 211.

15

BIOLOGICAL FUNCTION OF
IMMUNOGLOBULINS

OVERVIEW

The most obvious characteristic of the immunoglobulin molecule is the ability to combine specifically with antigen. However, immunoglobulin molecules have other properties. In this chapter we will discuss some of the other very interesting biological features of the immunoglobulin molecule as well as give some greater detail about the features of each of the classes of immunoglobulins.

FUNCTIONAL DOMAINS

We saw in the last chapter that antigen binding occurs in the Fab region and that the V regions and both H and L chains participate in the binding of antigen. Most of the other biological activities of the molecule are carried out in the Fc portion of the molecule. This division of labor within the molecule gives rise to the notion of *domains of function* within the immunoglobulin molecule. The V region thus contains the domain for the antigen-binding activity, and the C region contains the domain for the other biological activities of the molecule such as complement binding, skin fixation, and placental transport. Table 1 gives a summary of some of the physical and biological properties of the various immunoglobulin classes. In this chapter we will discuss properties of each class in greater detail, with emphasis on the function of the non-antigen-binding domain.

TABLE 1. PROPERTIES OF HUMAN IMMUNOGLOBULINS.

Class	IgG	IgM	IgA	IgD	IgE
H chains	γ	μ	α	δ	ϵ
L chains	κ,λ	κ,λ	κ,λ	κ,λ	κ,λ
Molecular weight	150,000	900,000	160,000	180,000	200,000
Number of subclasses	4	2	2	–	–
$S_{20,w}$	7	19	7,10,13, 15,17	6.5	–
Serum concentration, mg/ml	8–16	0.5–1.9	1.4–4.2	<0.4	<0.07
Complement fixation	+	+	–	–	
Placental passage	+	–	–	–	–
Seromucous secretions	–	–	+	–	–
Binding to mast cells	–	–	–	–	+

IgG

IgG is the most common class of immunoglobulin in normal serum, composing roughly 85 percent of the serum immunoglobulin in man. The normal concentration in human serum is between 8 and 16 mg/ml. IgG has a sedimentation coefficient of approximately 7s and a molecular weight of 150,000 to 170,000. The γ chain of human IgG has a molecular weight of approximately 53,000. The light chains have molecular weights of approximately 23,000. The ratio of k:λ chains is 3:1. The molecule contains roughly 3 percent carbohydrate which is attached to the Fc portion (with rare instances of carbohydrate on the light chain). From electron microscopic examination of antigen-antibody complexes plus recent X-ray diffraction studies the shape and dimension of the IgG molecule has been determined. Figure 1 is a model of the IgG molecule giving its dimensions.

All subclasses of IgG have antibody activity, but there is evidence in man that different antibody specificities are preferentially associated with different subclasses. For example, anti-tetanus antibody is associated with γ1 and anti-dextran antibody with γ2. There is heterogeneity in the skin-sensitizing ability of the human subclasses as well, γ2 lacking the ability to fix to skin. We have already noted that the Gm allotype is associated with IgG and that different Gm specificities are associated with different IgG subclasses.

IgG is the only immunoglobulin class which has the ability *to cross the placenta.* Maternal IgG but not IgM or IgA can be found in cord blood and in the fetus. Size of the molecule alone cannot be the

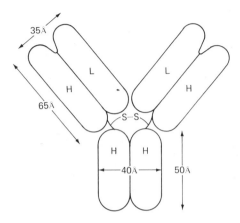

1

Scale diagram of a molecule of IgG. [From Green (1969). *Adv. Immunol.* **11, 1.]**

determining factor in placental transfer because serum IgA is approximately the same size as IgG. Furthermore, H chains cross the barrier, but L chains not linked to H chains do not. It appears that there is a structural basis for placental transfer in the Fc portion which allows the IgG molecule to be transported across the placenta and the other immunoglobulins not to be.

Each of the IgG subclasses also has a unique *catabolic rate* in a heterologous species. If the molecules are radiolabeled with iodine and injected into a rabbit, each of the human IgG subclasses will be eliminated from the circulation of the rabbit at a different but characteristic rate.

IgM

This class of immunoglobulin, which makes up 5 to 10 percent of serum immunoglobulin in normal serum, has a slightly faster electrophoretic mobility than those gamma globulins with a molecular weight of 170,000. Much of the structural work on IgM has been done with a pathological globulin derived from patients with *Waldenström macroglobulinemia*. Like patients with multiple myeloma, these individuals have a disorder of the lymphoid system in which certain immunoglobulin synthesizing and secreting cells proliferate at too rapid a rate. The result is a high level of IgM in the serum. Some of these Waldenström globulins appear to have antigen-binding (i.e., antibody) activity.

IgM molecules have a sedimentation coefficient of approximately 19s. The reported molecular weights range from 850,000 to 1,000,000 for human IgM. IgM molecules are approximately 12 percent carbohydrate, and the attachment of the carbohydrate to the μ chain seems to be at three points on the Fc fragment.

The IgM molecule is a *pentamer* of the monomeric units $(\mu_2 k_2)_5$ or $(\mu_2 \lambda_2)_5$ joined by disulfide bonds. The polymer can be dissociated into subunits called *IgMs* by thiol treatment under appropriate conditions. The monomeric unit has a molecular weight of approximately 180,000, and the monomers seem to reassociate into pentamers rather than random polymers. This is consistent with the circular shape of the molecule as determined by electron microscopic examination of antigen-antibody complexes. Figure 2 shows the dimensions and shape of the molecule.

A fragment called the J PROTEIN is found in polymerized IgM molecules and not in dissociated monomers. It is thought that this protein may have a role in joining the subunits into the polymer.

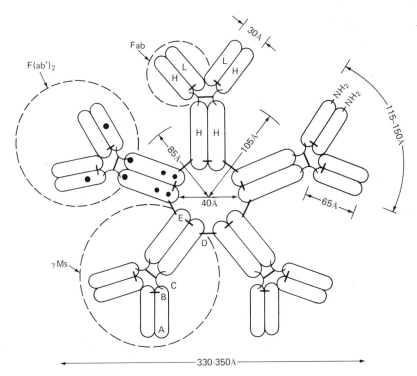

2

Scale diagram of IgM. [From Metzger (1970). *Adv. Immunol.* **12, 57.]**

The IgMs subunits can be dissociated into heavy and light chains (μ, κ, and λ) in the same manner as the IgG molecule. The μ chain has a molecular weight of 65,000 to 70,000, making it heavier than the γ chain of IgG. The light chains of IgM appear to be no different structurally or antigenically from those of IgG and the other classes of immunoglobulins.

Since monomeric units of immunoglobulin have two combining sites for antigen, it is of interest to determine the valence or number of antigen-binding sites for the pentamer. A Waldenström macroglobulin called IgM_{Lay} has been found which has the properties of *rheumatoid factor,* an IgM with antibody activity toward human IgG (i.e., human IgG acts as antigen and binds specifically to this human IgM which acts as antibody). Serum of patients with rheumatoid arthritis, an autoimmune disease, contains rheumatoid factor. Rheumatoid factor is found only in the IgM class of immunoglobulins. Data from this protein as well as serum IgM indicates that each molecule contains 10 identical combining sites per mole of IgM. Some studies with other antigens, however, show 5 combining sites (i.e., only 1 per monomer). It is not clear if there is steric hindrance of binding or if there is heterogeneity in the affinity of binding at the various sites on the pentameric molecule.

There is also some question about the relative *avidity* (firmness of binding) in IgG and IgM antibody molecules. Studies with some antigens, e.g., toxins, enzymes, some bacteria, and viruses, indicate that IgM is less avid than IgG. Other studies show that they are the same, and as is so often the case in immunology, others show that IgM is more avid than IgG.

There is agreement on the fact that IgM is more efficient than IgG, causing the *agglutination* of erythrocytes. Some studies show that IgM anti-erythrocyte antibody is 100 times more efficient at hemagglutination (see Appendix I) than is IgG anti-erythrocyte antibody, meaning that it takes 100 times more molecules of IgG than IgM to achieve a certain degree of agglutination. This points up the fact that assays for antibody activity which rely on agglutination of erythrocytes or bacteria tend to favor the detection of IgM over IgG.

The *fixation of complement* is also carried out more efficiently by IgM than by IgG. The complement system is a complex one of 11 serum proteins which are activated in sequence, very much like the proteins involved in blood clotting. The initiation of the "complement cascade" occurs when the initial component of complement reacts with the Fc portion of an antibody molecule which has combined with antigen. Erythrocyte antigens are most commonly used in complement studies because lysis of the cell is the final result, and this is an easily measured reaction. Complement will not react with uncombined antibody or antigen. It has been demonstrated that for the initial interaction to occur a doublet of IgG molecules is needed. This means that two IgG molecules spaced close to each other must have reacted with antigens in the cell membrane of the erythrocyte. But, because IgM is a pentamer, the requirement for a "doublet" is fulfilled within the individual molecule, and so only one molecule of bound IgM is needed to initiate the complement cascade. Because thiol breaks the disulfide bonds and disrupts the relationship between the monomers, treatment of IgM with thiol reagents lowers the efficiency of complement binding and activation. Many assays for antibody concentration in a serum are done with the addition of a thiol reagent, mercaptoethanol, which reduces the intermonomer disulfides, and thus the pentameric structure is lost. The reduced molecule loses its high efficiency of complement binding, and both *mercaptoethanol-sensitive* (usually 19s and IgM) and *mercaptoethanol-resistant* (usually 7s and IgG) antibodies are determined. It is again to be noted that complement-binding assays favor the detection of IgM over IgG.

IgA

The notion of *local immunity* in some infectious diseases has been known for many years. For example, immunity to cholera correlates with the titer of antibodies in the feces (termed *coproantibodies*) rather than the serum antibody titer. Similarly, the concentration of diphtheria antitoxin is high in saliva. Antibodies which are important in resistance to infection and are found in external secretions have been noted in many diseases; no doubt they compose a significant means of resistance to infection. The dominant class of antibody in external secretions is IgA, the so-called *secretory immunoglobulin*.

IgA is found in serum and secretions of the parotid, submaxillary, and lacrimal glands, in nasal, tracheobronchial, gastric, and seminal fluid, and in urine as well as in colostrum. In serum the molecular weight of IgA is approximately 170,000, whereas secretory IgA and colostral IgA have molecular weights closer to 380,000. These weights correspond to sedimentation coefficients of approximately 7s and 11s. Polymers of 16 to 20s also occur in secretions. The serum concentration of IgA is approximately 1 to 4 mg/ml.

The H chain of IgA, the α chain, is the same for both serum and colostral molecules. The molecular weight of the α chain is approximately 65,000, thus making it larger than the γ chain of IgG which has a molecular weight of 53,000 in man. Human α chain does not carry the Gm allotype. The light chains, κ and λ, are no different than those of other immunoglobulin molecules. The light chains of some myeloma protein IgA have been shown to be connected by disulfide bonds, thus placing them in close proximity, but this is not true of all IgA molecules.

It is generally accepted that a unique structure, the SECRETORY PIECE (SP), is associated with the IgA molecule which allows it to be secreted. Secretory piece has been identified in alkaline urea gels of IgA as a unique fast-moving cationic band. In rabbit colostral IgA which has been reduced and alkylated, a similar band, called TRANS-PORT (T), has been observed. The secretory piece is of great interest but the way it is linked to the IgA molecule is not yet clear. Data showing both covalent and noncovalent linking is available. The molecular weight of isolated SP is approximately 50,000 to 60,000, and the molecule may consist of two subunits, each with a molecular weight of 25,000, linked by disulfide bonds. SP probably is linked to the α chain. It has been suggested that SP is synthesized in epithelial cells and added to the IgA molecule as it is transported across the mucous membrane. The J protein is also associated with IgA in its polymeric form.

IgD

The first indication of this fourth class of human immunoglobulin resulted from the study of an unusual human myeloma protein. The concentration in the serum of IgD is very low, approximately 3 to 40 μg/ml (note that this unit of measure is *microgram;* IgG, IgM, and IgA concentrations were given in *milligrams*). The fact that the concentration in serum is so low makes study of the molecule very difficult. Study of the molecule from serum is further complicated by the fact that IgD is a very labile molecule. It is much more sensitive to proteolysis and heat than the other immunoglobulin classes, and proteolytic enzymes in serum may be sufficient to fragment the molecule during isolation procedures.

The molecular weight of IgD is approximately 180,000. The δ chain has a molecular weight of 60,000 to 70,000. There is approximately 12 percent carbohydrate which is associated with the δ chain, although there is a possibility that a small percent of IgD molecules has some carbohydrate on the light chains.

The apparent biological function of IgD has recently been established. IgD is found to be present on the surface membranes of large numbers of human peripheral lymphocytes. It is often found in association with IgM on the same cell. When immunoglobulin was isolated from the surfaces of mouse lymphocytes, a unique immuno-globulin was found (by molecular weight and mobility in polyacrylamide gels). This mouse immunoglobulin has physical properties similar to human IgD and is tentatively being called IgD (there is as yet no mouse myeloma secreting IgD). It may be that because of its membrane-bound position IgD serves as the immunoglobulin receptor for antigen on the lymphocyte surface (see Chapter 10).

IgE

IgE is also a minor component of normal serum, having a concentration in human serum of approximately 1 μg/ml in healthy individuals. IgE has a molecular weight of approximately 190,000. The ϵ chain has an approximate molecular weight of 72,500. IgE does not seem to be a secretory immunoglobulin, its concentration being low in nasal and mucal secretions. Some women show a high concentration of IgE in colostrum, while others do not.

IgE levels are greatly increased in asthma and hay fever patients, the serum concentration being about 20 times higher than normal. Children suffering from various atopic diseases show elevated IgE levels. There are no changes in IgE levels in patients with some other immunological disorders, e.g., rheumatoid arthritis, systemic lupus erythematosis, and ulcerative colitis. Certain infectious diseases such as pneumonia and hepatitis also do not seem to cause elevated IgE levels.

IgE is considered the *reaginic* antibody. Reagins are antibodies against allergens which are involved in immediate (reaginic) hypersensitivity or allergy, as opposed to cell-mediated (delayed or tuberculin) hypersensitivity. Reaginic antibodies have the ability to bind firmly to tissues. When the allergen is introduced by skin contact or inhalation, the combination of reagin and allergin on the surface of cells, primarily mast cells, results in the liberation by those cells of pharmacologically active substances. These agents may induce vasodilation, smooth muscle contraction, or increased vascular permeability to shock organs, leading to the manifestation of asthma, eczema, etc.

EVOLUTION OF IMMUNOGLOBULINS

All species of vertebrates appear to be able to make immunoglobulins. The most primitive, well-studied, species is the lamprey (a cyclostome). Lamprey immunoglobulin is heterogeneous, containing 7s and 14s molecules. The molecule has a chain structure, but the H and L chains do not seem to be linked by disulfide bridges. The L chain has a molecular weight of 24,000, similar to a mammalian L chain. The H chain has a molecular weight of 70,000, similar to a mammalian μ chain. The interesting feature of the chains is that there seems to be no antigenic difference between them. The same is true of elasmobranch immunoglobulins. The shark has L chains of approximately 20,000 molecular weight and H chains of 70,000 with no antigenic differences between them. The electrophoretic mobility, carbohydrate content, and molecular weight of shark H chain seem to be similar to mammalian μ chain. The chains of elasmobranch immunoglobulins are joined by disulfide bonds, as are the amphibia, but there are antigenic differences between the 7s and 19s immunoglobulins of amphibia.

Because of the absence of Bence Jones proteins and other myeloma proteins in the more primitive forms, detailed studies of sequence have not been possible. In mammals where sequence or peptide maps are readily available, some interesting facts emerge about the evolutionary relationship between immunoglobulins. When human and mouse Bence Jones proteins are compared, the similarities between human κ and mouse κ chains are found to be greater than the similarities between human κ and human λ chains. Thus the intraspecies homology between different classes of L chains is not as great as the interspecies homology between chains of the

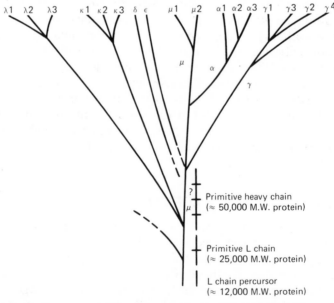

3

Evolution of immunoglobin genes. [From Grey (1969). *Adv. Immunol.* 10, 51.]

same class. Kappa chains of different species have more homology of amino acid sequence than do κ and λ chains of the same species.

By examination of the available data on structural and sequence homology, an evolutionary tree of immunoglobulin genes has been constructed and is shown in Figure 3. It can be seen that the primitive L chain probably gave rise to the primitive H chain (which was probably μ-like) by gene duplication. This occurred ca. 400,000,-000 years ago when the vertebrates were emerging. Two hundred million years ago, when the amphibians were emerging, the classes of immunoglobulins arose. The subclasses have probably arisen more recently by duplication and deletion.

SUMMARY

1. IgG is the Ig found in highest concentration in the serum and is a monomer.
2. IgM is a pentamer. The subunits are joined by the J protein. IgM is extremely efficient in C fixation and agglutination. Antibody reactions carried out by IgM are susceptible to mercaptoethanol treatment.
3. IgA is a secretory immunoglobulin. A structure called the secretory piece is responsible for secretion of the molecule from epithelial tissue.
4. IgD is found in extremely low concentration in the serum. It is found on the surface of B-cells and may play a role as an antigen receptor on these cells.
5. IgE is the antibody associated with allergy. IgE has the property of fixing to tissues so that when it reacts with antigen (allergen) it causes the release of vasoactive compounds from cells.

READINGS

REVIEWS

Green, N. M. (1969). Electron microscopy of the immunoglobulins, *Adv. Immunol.* **11**, 1.

Metzger, H. (1970) Structure and function of γM macroglobulins, *Adv. Immunol.* **12**, 57.

Bennich, H., and Johansson, S. G. O. (1971). Structure and function of human immunoglobulin E, *Adv. Immunol.* **13**, 1.

Spiegelberg, H. L. (1974). Biological activities of immunoglobulins of different classes and subclasses, *Adv. Immunol.* **19**, 259.

Lamm, M. E. (1976). Cellular aspects of immunoglobulin A, *Adv. Immunol.* **22**, 223.

Koshland, M. E. (1975). Structure and function of the J chain, *Adv. Immunol.* **20**, 41.

16

GENERATION OF DIVERSITY

OVERVIEW

One of the most intriguing features of the immune response is the fact that an animal can produce different antibody molecules which can react specifically with a vast number of antigens. The number of antibody specificities which an animal can generate is generally thought to be of the order of 10^6, although the number could be either much higher or much lower. In this chapter we will discuss some of the possible mechanisms by which this great diversity can be generated as well as consider the fact that in accounting for the diversity any theory must also account for much nondiversity or "commonness" between antibody molecules of different specificities.

STRUCTURAL BASIS OF SPECIFICITY

There is little doubt that the specificity of antigen binding resides in the primary structure (the linear arrangement of amino acids) of the antibody molecule. Secondary and tertiary structures are also a function of primary structure since the folding and shape of protein molecules have been clearly demonstrated to depend upon the sequence of amino acids. When antibody molecules are treated in a manner to disrupt all noncovalent interactions and break all disulfide bonds, the ability to bind with antigen is lost. When the molecules are allowed to spontaneously return to their native configuration in the absence of the unfolding agent and antigen, they regain the ability to bind antigen. Since the configuration to which they return is dependent on the primary structure, it follows that the specificity of antigen binding arises from the specificity of the sequence of the amino acids.

We know that the binding domain of the immunoglobulin molecule is in the Fab region and that there are enough possible unique amino acid sequences in the V region to account for over 10^6 specificities. This is the structural basis of diversity. Since the primary structure of a protein is a function of the linear array of the nucleotides in the DNA, it follows that if there are 10^6 different sequences of amino acids there must be 10^6 sequences of DNA coding for them. It is also known that an individual cell produces antibody of only one specificity, and so we must be able to account for the fact that an animal can make antibodies of 10^6 different specificities (and therefore have the genetic information for these specificities) but have the information packaged in such a manner that an antibody-producing cell synthesizes only one of the 10^6 specificities. This raises the question of whether each cell has the ability to produce antibodies with all the specificities but is expressing only one of them or whether the packaging is done by somehow distributing the genetic information for only one specificity to a cell.

GENES CODING FOR IMMUNOGLOBULIN MOLECULES

The question must also be answered of whether the information for all the responses a member of a species can make is transmitted from parent to offspring via the sperm and egg (the germ cells) or whether a few basic antibody specificity genes are transmitted and then the animal generates the entire body of genetic information from these few genes in somatic cells. These are obviously profound questions and, as with all such profound questions, they are difficult to answer. The approach which immunologists have taken is to compare sequences of amino acids of different immunoglobulins as a means of determining the nature of the genetic information. The number of defined structural features in immunoglobulin molecules which are found in all members of the species is the minimal number of genes required to code for the immunoglobulins which the members of the species can make. Any of the structures may have variants, and this is a measure of the number of alleles for a given gene.

We shall first consider the data which allows an estimate of the minimal number of genes for H- and L-chain V and C regions. Then we will examine the theories for the packaging of the genes for antibody specificities.

Constant-Region Genes

We already know that class and subclass of immunoglubulins are determined by structural components in the C region of the H chains. In man, it will be remembered, the Gm allotype is found on the C_H chain, and so a set of genetic markers is available for study of this chain. Because the number of discrete structural entities defines the minimum number of genes, the number of subclasses of an immunoglobulin can be used to determine the minimal number of C_H region genes. A normal individual synthesizes all classes and subclasses of immunoglobulins. Since in man there are four subclasses of IgG (IgG 1, 2, 3, 4), two for IgA, two for IgM, and one each for IgD and IgE, every normal human must have a minimum of 10 genes coding for C_H regions. Similarly, for C_L there is one for k and two for λ, which means a minimum of three C_L genes.

Variable-Region Genes

Analysis of amino acid sequences has resulted in classifying immunoglobulins into *families* on the basis of similarities of structure. In man there are three κ families and four λ families in the V region. For the κ chain there are three genes which code for the Vκ region (VκI, VκII, and VκIII), but only one gene for the Cκ region (Cκ). This means that any of the three Vκ genes can be associated with a single structural C gene. Human λ chains have four Vλ genes (VλI, VλII, VλIII, and VλIV), and these can be associated with the two C genes.

Genealogy of Light Chains

A hypothetical genealogic tree of human V_L families is seen in Figure 1. This genealogic tree indicates the hypothetical minimum number of genetic events (base substitutions, insertions or deletions, and gene duplications) which would be required to convert a primordial V_L gene (level A of Figure 1) to a present-day V gene (level F of the figure). Since antibodies would have unique stretches of amino acid sequences in their V region, the fact that there exist families of related structural V regions (i.e., areas of similar structure) must mean that sequence diversity for antibody specificity is found along with the commonness. Thus, any theory must explain the retention of family traits (commonness) and the generation of antibody diversity (variability) within the family.

Two genes, one polypeptide chain

We have already established the fact that there are multiple germ-line Vκ genes (VκI, VκII, and VκIII) and that there is but a

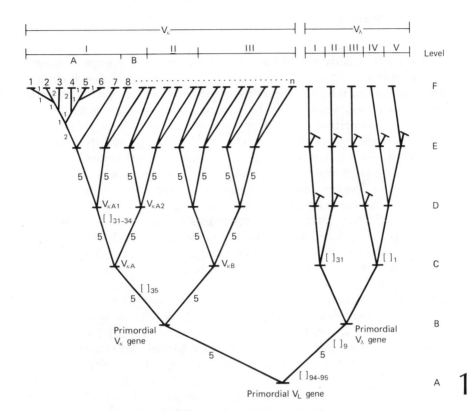

A hypothetical genealogical tree for human V_L regions. A genealogical tree is constructed from a set of proteins (numbers at level F) by generating a series of ancestral or nodal sequences (levels E, D, C, etc.) using a minimum number of base substitutions, sequence insertions or deletions, and gene duplications. The genetic events responsible for generating this genealogic pattern could occur, in part, during somatic differentiation (somatic theory) or entirely during the evolution of the species (germ line theory). $I, II,$ and III represent distinct branches (subgroups) on the tree. [From Hood, et al. (1975). Ann. Rev. Genetics 9, 301. Copyright © 1975 by Annual Reviews, Inc. All rights reserved.]

single $C\kappa$ germ-line gene. Thus any $V\kappa$ region can associate with the single $C\kappa$ region to produce a completed kappa chain. This being so, there must be a mechanism which unites either the two genes or their products. In either case, we find the interesting situation of two genes coding for a single polypeptide chain, the completed kappa chain in this case. This is in contrast with the dictum of one gene, one enzyme or polypeptide chain.

ANTIBODY DIVERSITY

Site

We have already stated that the variability in sequence responsible for antibody specificity is in the V region of the H and L chains and that as many as 10^6 sequences must be coded for. The V regions, as we have just shown, can be grouped into families according to sequence similarities within the variable region. Where then is the site of diversity for all the antibody specificities which must be generated? As we saw in Chapter 14, there are stretches of amino acids whose sequences are similar in the V region and areas where there is no "commonness," i.e., areas of high variability. If one compares the sequences of 10 κ chains belonging to a given Vκ family (and by definition having some sequences in common), one will find "hot spots" of variability as well as variations in length of the chains which are the result of deletions or gaps. It is in these "hot spots" and gaps that we believe lies the structural basis of diversity.

Germ-line vs. Somatic Mechanisms

The question now becomes, considering the above, what are the mechanisms by which the diversity for antibody specificity is generated but the commonness of the families retained? Two major classes of theories attempt to account for the facts. One theory, the GERM-LINE THEORY, argues that the information for all the specificities to which the species can respond is transmitted from parent to offspring in the germ cells (sperm and egg). Thus, according to this theory, *all* the genes in level F of Figure 1 are transmitted to each generation from its parents and in some manner packaged by the offspring into somatic cells.

An alternate theory, the SOMATIC MUTATION THEORY, argues that a limited number of genes are transmitted in the germ line. This number would correspond to some level between C and E in Figure 1. The theory argues that this small number of genes is transmitted in the germ cells and then the genes undergo mutational events in somatic cells such that the number of specificities required (*ca.* 10^6) for level F is attained in the somatic cells. A variation of this theory, the SOMATIC RECOMBINATION THEORY, states that a limited (but perhaps large) number of genes are transmitted in the germ line but that these genes, instead of mutating (changing DNA bases), undergo translocations (reshuffling of the order of stretches of the DNA) in the somatic cells, thus giving rise to the large number of genes needed for antibody diversity.

Proponents of the germ-line theory argue that the genealogy studies show that a significant number of "genetic events" must occur to move from one level of Figure 1 to another. To retain the commonness of the families while still generating the diversity of the antibody-combining sites would require a large number of parallel genetic events or a sequential series of mutational events. This number is very large, and an ad hoc series of events must be invented to account for the molecules found at level F. The germ-line theory, they argue, does not require such ad hoc mechanisms since all the genes for all the specificities are always present.

A major argument which the proponents of the somatic theories raise against the germ-line theory is one of "genetic drift." If 10^6 specificities are required, only a small number of them may be used during the animal's lifetime. That is to say, an animal may or may not be confronted with a given antigen. If not confronted, the gene for that antibody specificity has had no selective pressures placed on it during that generation. Considering the wide array of specificities to which animals can respond, it is conceivable that large numbers of genes will not be called upon during the lifetime of the animal. An unselected gene can therefore spontaneously mutate and "drift" and thus be lost to the offspring of a given animal. If this were to occur, the responses of the species would not be as uniform as they are.

SUMMARY

1. The structural basis of antibody specificity is the sequence of amino acids in the antigen-binding site of the hypervariable regions.

2. By calculating the number of regions, subregions, and allotypic determinants for an Ig chain, it is possible to calculate the minimal number of genes needed to code for that chain.

3. Variable regions can be grouped into families based on similarity of sequence. By grouping these families, a hypothetical genealogical tree which traces a primordial V_1 gene to present-day diversity can be constructed.

4. The immunoglobulin chain is coded for by more than one gene but yields one polypeptide chain. This leads to the idea of two genes–one polypeptide.

5. Two major theories for the generation of diversity are germ line and somatic variation. Germ line argues that all the genes for antibody specificity are passed through the sperm and egg. Somatic variation argues that a small number of genes are passed from generation to generation as germ cells but these undergo mutation or recombination when they are in somatic cells.

READINGS

REVIEWS

Hood, L., and Talmage, D. W. (1970). Mechanism of antibody diversity: germ line basis for variability, *Science* **168,** 325.

Gally, J. A. and Edelman, G. M. (1970). Somatic translocation of antibody genes, *Nature (London)*, **227**, 341.

Cohn, M. (1974). A rationale for ordering the data on antibody diversification, in *Progress in Immunology* II, L. Brent and J. Holborow (eds.), New York, Elsevier, 261.

(Three very good reviews giving the germ line and somatic viewpoints of generation of diversity.)

Jerne, N. K. (1971). The somatic generation of immune recognition, *Europ. J. Immunol.* **1**, 1. (A very creative attempt to give a cellular basis for diversity.)

Hood, L., Campbell, J. H., and Elgin, S. C. A. (1975). The organization, expression and evolution of antibody genes and other multigene families, *Annu. Rev. Gene.* **9**, 305. (An excellent review of possible genetic and nongenetic mechanisms for generation of diversity.)

IV

REGULATION OF THE IMMUNE RESPONSE

Up to now we have developed the idea that lymphocytes react with antigen through antigen-specific receptors at their surface. For the interaction to result in either an antibody or a cell-mediated response, there must be interaction between helper and effector cells. A central tenet of the clonal selection theory is that a small number of these lymphocytes in the normal population are preprogrammed to respond to an antigen. This means that the small number of precursors of effector cells is induced to proliferate and differentiate into functional effector cells, resulting in large numbers of effector cells in a short time. In this section we will examine some of the experiments which show that there is antigen-induced clonal expansion of effector cells. Specific interaction with antigen results in proliferation of specific cells but also a change in the population, called the maturation of the immune response. This term refers to the changes which occur in the character of the cells undergoing an immune response once it is initiated. Early antibody in a response is IgM, but there is a shift to IgG.

One class of T-cells can act as a suppressor of immune responses. This cell is called the suppressor T-cell (Ts). It appears in a variety of situations and can be either antigen specific or nonspecific. Some suppress by cell contact and some by soluble factors. It is becoming clear that suppressor cells may play a very important or even central role in the regulation of the immune response.

The ability to respond to certain antigens is under genetic control. While this fact is to be expected, the discovery that many of the genes which control the immune responses are located in the major histocompatibility complex was not only surprising but has opened the way to further understanding of the immune response.

It is possible to experimentally induce a state of specific nonresponsiveness to an antigen. This is called immune tolerance and serves as a model for studying tolerance to self-antigens. The mechanism of tolerance to self and foreign antigens is not known. Possibly specific clones are eliminated in tolerance, or they may be present but unable to function. The suppressor T-cell may play a role in this checking of autoreactive cells.

17

PROLIFERATION AND MATURATION

OVERVIEW

The essence of the immune response is the activation of a small number of precursor cells and their expansion into a population of functional effector cells. In this chapter we will show that antigen induces proliferation in those cells which are committed to respond to the specific antigen. This means that during a response there is clonal expansion of cells with specific antigen reactivity.

The properties of the antibody which the B-cells produce also change during the course of a response. The first antibodies produced in a primary response are IgM, but there is a shift to IgG synthesis during the primary response. During the secondary response almost all the antibody produced is IgG. Among the 7s antibody molecules a change in binding affinity also occurs during the course of the response. The change in affinity is due to the selection by antigen of cells able to produce high-affinity antibody. These cells preferentially react with antigen and are thus preferentially induced to proliferate. Antigen can thus be visualized as selecting to proliferate only cells with specific antigen-binding receptors and also as preferentially selecting those with high-affinity receptors.

PROLIFERATION IN THE IMMUNE RESPONSE

Primary and Secondary Responses

The introduction of antigen either *in vivo* or *in vitro* results in antibody production with kinetics typical of those seen in Figure 1.

209

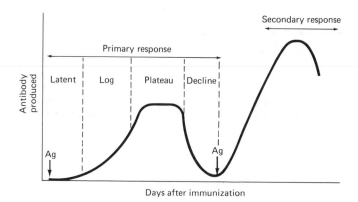

Kinetics of primary and secondary antibody responses.

For a short period of time after antigen is introduced, no detectable antibody is synthesized. This period is called the LATENT PHASE.[1] After the latent phase antibody formation occurs at an exponential rate. This period is called the LOG PHASE. After the log phase there is a period of equilibrium with no net increase or decrease in antibody synthesis which is called the PLATEAU PHASE. This phase is followed by a drop in antibody formation which is called the DECLINE PHASE.

The first curve in Figure 1 represents the antibody response of an animal to the first contact with an antigen. This is called the PRIMARY RESPONSE. If the same antigen is reintroduced, the kinetics seen in the second curve in Figure 1 are obtained. This is called the SECONDARY RESPONSE. In the secondary response there is a much shorter latent period, and the magnitude of the response (the amount of antibody produced or the number of antibody-producing cells) is greater. We will see later in this chapter that the class of immunoglobulin also changes in primary and secondary responses.

Antigen-Induced Proliferation of Effector Cells

The exponential increase in antibody-forming cells after the introduction of antigen strongly suggests that effector cells or their precursors are proliferating. This can be readily demonstrated by pulsing a culture with radiolabeled nucleotides and showing by autoradiography that the label appears in the DNA of the antibody-forming cell. The essence of clonal expansion is that antigen in some manner induces a specific cell to proliferate. The clones of cells

---

[1]The kinetic curve in Figure 1 is so similar to a bacterial growth curve that the phases of the curve have been given the same names.

expanded in this manner have been "selected" in an evolutionary sense. There is good evidence that the precursor of the antibody-forming cell is not a proliferating cell *before* contact with antigen but becomes one after antigenic stimulation.

Two kinds of experiments have shown that the precursor of the antibody-forming cells are not proliferating before the introduction of antigen. The first uses drugs which inhibit mitosis. For example, the drug vinblastine irreversibly inhibits proliferation of cells which enter into mitosis. Resting cells are unaffected by the drug, and only cells in mitosis are inhibited from further proliferation. When vinblastine was injected several days *before antigen,* it had no effect on the number of antibody-forming cells produced. When it was given shortly *after antigen,* it abolished the generation of antibody-forming cells. Since the drug can affect only cells in mitosis and has no effect when given several days before antigen, this argues that the precursor of the antibody-forming cell was not in mitosis before antigen was introduced. The fact that the drug abolished the response when it was given shortly after antigen argues that antigen had induced proliferation of effector cells.

The second kind of experiment uses tritiated thymidine of high specific activity to answer the same question. Thymidine labeled with tritium of extremely high specific activity, when incorporated into the DNA of a cell, releases enough energy in the nucleus to irreversibly damage the proliferative capacity of the cell. This is called "tritium suicide." When a tritium suicide experiment is performed on cultures of spleen cells before or after the introduction of antigen, it is found that adding the tritiated thymidine of high specific activity before antigen has no effect on an antibody response. However, when added after antigen, it inhibits further antibody production. Both of these kinds of experiments are diagrammed in Figure 2.

The proliferation induced by antigen is specific. Normal responses to antigen X are obtained if antigen Y is added to a culture and the culture is then treated with tritiated thymidine of high specific activity before antigen X is added. Since we know that such tritiated thymidine has no effect before addition of antigen, this experiment argues that only the *specific* precursor cell is induced to proliferate by antigen.

Antigen-Induced Proliferation of Helper Cells

If neonatally thymectomized mice are reconstituted with a graft of thymus lobes placed under the kidney capsule, the immune function of these mice is restored. If the thymus lobe is derived from an animal which has a marker such as the T6T6 chromosome, it is possible to

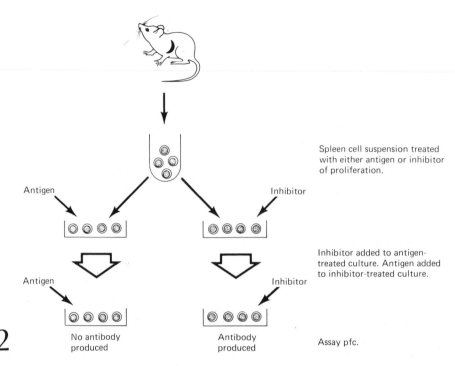

Spleen cell suspension treated
with either antigen or inhibitor
of proliferation.

Antigen   Inhibitor

Inhibitor added to antigen-
treated culture. Antigen added
to inhibitor-treated culture.

Antigen   Inhibitor

No antibody   Antibody
produced   produced   Assay pfc.

2

Inhibition of proliferation after antigen stimulation inhibits antibody response. [After Syeklocha *et al.* (1966). *J. Immunol.* 96, 472, and Dutton and Mishell (1967). *Cold Spring Harbor Symposium on Quantitative Biology*, 32, 407.]

identify and count these cells in the spleen and lymph nodes at later times. It can be shown in this manner that after antigenic stimulation there is a transient but well-defined increase in the number of these cells. Furthermore, it can be shown that T-cells have an increased uptake of exogenously added tritiated thymidine after introduction of antigen and also that the number of helper cells in a population increases after antigenic stimulation. We saw in Chapter 8 that the helper cell in cell-mediated responses is probably the cell which undergoes an MLR. Taken together, this data argues that helper cells are induced to proliferate by antigen. Whether proliferation is in some manner connected to the way they exert their helper function is not known. It does show, however, that helper cell population is expanded by antigen contact.

MATURATION OF THE ANTIBODY RESPONSE

During the course of the antibody response a series of changes occurs in the characteristics of the antibody molecules which are produced. Both the *class* and the *affinity* of the antibody change. These changes are termed the MATURATION of the antibody response.

Shift of Ig Class

One of the most striking changes which occurs during an antibody response is the change of the *class* of the antibody being produced. During a primary antibody response to most antigens there is a shift from predominantly IgM production early in the response to predominantly IgG production later in the response. Figure 3 shows a typical curve in which total antibody, 19s, and 7s antibody are plotted against time in a primary and secondary response. Note that the total antibody reaches a level and maintains that level during the plateau phase of the response. A shift from IgM antibody to IgG occurs during the course of the response.

Methods of Detecting IgM and IgG Antibody

It was shown in Chapter 15 that IgM, being a pentamer, is more efficient in lysis and agglutination reactions than IgG. Accordingly, when equal numbers of IgM and IgG molecules are compared in assays using hemolysis or agglutination, the IgM molecules show more activity. But because IgM is a pentamer in which the

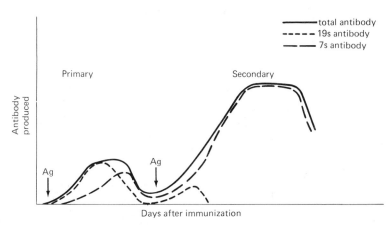

Change in class of antibody during a primary and a secondary response.

monomeric units are joined by disulfide bonds, the molecule is readily split into its monomers by reducing agents such as mercaptoethanol (ME). The monomers have activity roughly comparable with IgG so that when a sample of serum which contains IgM antibody is compared before and after reduction with mercaptoethanol, the titer is found to be greatly reduced after treatment. In contrast, because IgG is already a monomer, treatment with mercaptoethanol has no effect on the titer.

Because of this reduction of titer after 2-ME treatment of IgM, antibody titers are often expressed as mercaptoethanol-sensitive (MES) or mercaptoethanol-resistant (MER) antibody. MES antibody is equated with 19s (IgM), and MER is equated with 7s (IgG).

To determine if a plaque-forming cell is producing IgM or IgG antibodies, a method called the *indirect plaque assay* is used (Figure 4). In this method the antibody-forming cell produces IgG which diffuses and reacts with the RBC in the medium. Since IgG has low efficiency of lysis, a plaque does not develop when complement is added. However, if an antibody directed against the IgG molecule is then added, this anti-IgG reacts with the IgG on the RBC, and lysis occurs in the presence of complement.

Cellular Basis of the 19s to 7s Shift

The cellular mechanism of the 19s to 7s shift is not known. The change in antibody class could be due to two B-cell populations each synthesizing and secreting a single class of antibody but appearing at different times after antigenic stimulation, or it could be due to the same cell line producing 19s and then shifting to produce 7s antibody. Considering the structure of the combining site on the immunoglobulin molecule, the latter explanation means that a set of V_H and V_L genes is being associated first with genes coding for the μ chain and then for the γ chain.

To determine if a single cell is able to produce more than one class of immunoglobulin, Nossal and his co-workers have used a microdrop technique in which it has been possible to study the class of antibody produced by a single cell. Single lymphocytes producing anti-*Salmonella* antibody were cultured in individual droplets. The fluid from each droplet was then divided into two droplets, and mercaptoethanol was added to one of the drops. The ability of the antibodies in the two droplets to agglutinate the bacterial antigens was then tested. In 17 of 123 droplets (almost 14 percent) there were cells producing both MES and MER antibody. Using the same microdrop method but adding anti-μ or anti-γ antibodies instead of mercaptoethanol, the same group has found that 14 of 900 (only 1.5 percent)

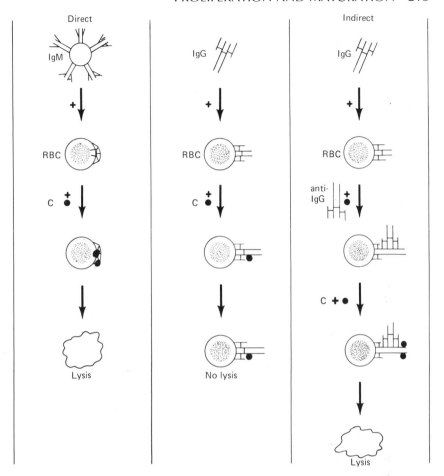

Direct ... **Indirect**

Lysis — No lysis — Lysis

4

Detection of IgM and IgG antibodies by direct and indirect hemolytic methods.

of the droplets were producing both classes. The method is very sensitive, and the approximately 2 percent of the cells found to be producing both classes could be a real reflection of cells undergoing the shifting process. This would argue for a single cell producing both classes.

There is also data which argues that IgM- and IgG-producing cells are derived from *separate* precursors. This data, obtained by re-populating lethally irradiated animals with limiting dilutions of cells and determining if IgM and IgG producers are found with the same frequency, shows that the two classes appear at different frequencies, and from this it is argued that they arise from separate precursor cells.

Perhaps the most convincing data to show that a molecular mechanism exists for the same cell to produce IgG and IgM comes from data on a human myeloma which synthesizes and secretes both μ and γ chains. From idiotypic markers it was determined that the same cell was producing both classes of immunoglobulin. When the amino acid sequences of the V regions were determined, it was found that the V regions for both the IgG and IgM were identical. This is important because it indicates that there exists a mechanism whereby the V region genes can be fitted to at least two sets of C region genes.

From all this it is clear that the question of the cellular basis of the class shift in antibody synthesis is far from resolved.

CHANGE IN ANTIBODY AFFINITY AFTER IMMUNIZATION

Another change which occurs during the maturation of the immune response is an *increase in affinity* of the antibody produced. Antigen reacts specifically with antibody to form antigen-antibody complexes, and like most chemical reactions the antigen-antibody interaction can be described in thermodynamic terms. AFFINITY is a measure of the strength of the union between the two reactants. More energy is required to separate a complex formed between high-affinity antibody and antigen than to separate one formed with low-affinity antibody. The strength of the union is usually given in terms of the equilibrium constant (K) in units of liters per mole. A high K value indicates a high affinity. Since K is inversely related to standard free energy change ($\Delta F°$), a high-affinity union (high K) has a low $\Delta F°$. AVIDITY is a less precise, nonthermodynamic, term which also refers to the strength of the union between antigen and antibody. Avidity is usually measured by biological rather than chemical means.

When the antibody in the serum of an animal at any time after challenge with an antigen is examined closely, it is found to be *heterogeneous for binding affinity*. Fractionation of the antiserum can be carried out by adding small amounts of antigen, collecting the precipitate, and determining the binding constant of the precipitated fraction. Repetition of this procedure shows that there can be as much as a thousandfold difference in affinity between the fractions precipitated. The binding constant for the unfractionated serum, of course, reflects an average of all the affinities. The average affinity of the serum increases during the course of immunization.

By use of equilibrium dialysis it has been shown that when low or moderate doses of antigen are used for immunization, the average intrinsic association constant (K_0) of the antibody produced increases with time after immunization. Typical data from such an experiment is seen in Figure 5. The fact that the change in affinity did not occur at high-antigen doses will be used later in constructing a theory to explain the maturation of the response. When the maturation of the immune response is studied with protein antigens, similar results are obtained. For example, the avidity of anti-BSA for BSA rises progressively during immunization. In these experiments the avidity of the BSA-anti-BSA complex is determined by the amount of dissociation of the complex in excess BSA at various times after immunization.

Studies with toxin-anti-toxin systems also have shown a greater avidity later in the response than early. Particulate antigens such as bacteriophage and heterologous erythrocytes give similar results. There are some exceptions, however; the antibody against pneumococcus polysaccharide antigen in the rabbit does not change avidity during the course of the response. The structure of the antigen or the manner in which it is processed by the animal may be of great importance in the maturation of the response. As a general rule, thymus-independent antigens show less change in affinity and avidity than do thymus-dependent antigens. These antigens also give less IgG, which is the class in which the greatest increase in affinity occurs.

The change in affinity seems to occur primarily in the IgG class of immunoglobulins. Studies which have examined the change in affin-

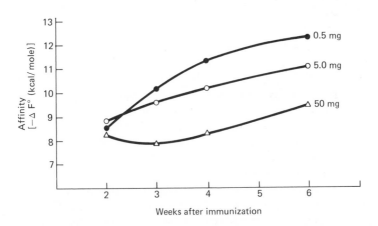

Change in affinity of antibody after immunization with various doses of antigen. (Adapted from Siskind *et al.* (1968). *J. Exp. Med.* **127**, 55.)

ity in IgM for the most part find that the affinity remains constant during the course of the immunization, although some studies have shown that the affinity of IgM rises. The differences between various reports may be due to the antigens used and the methods of measuring affinity or avidity. IgA antibody does not seem to have a change in affinity. In the guinea pig the change in affinity was observed to occur in both subclasses of IgG (γ_1 and γ_2).

Clonal Nature of Increased Affinity

The increase in affinity seen in antibody responses can be due to changes in the molecules which a cell is producing or changes in the population of cells. Since there is some evidence that a cell can change from IgM to IgG synthesis, one might reasonably think that it could also change the affinity of the molecules it produces. On the other hand, one might also reasonably postulate that a cell produces antibody of one affinity and cells which produce the highest affinity antibody increase in number during the response. This would mean that the affinity of the antibody produced by cells is clonal.

To test this question, a modification of the *in vitro* focus-forming assay (Chapter 12) was carried out. The experiment is seen in Figure 6. Irradiated mice were repopulated with low numbers of spleen cells from primed mice. One day later the spleen was removed, and cut into fragments, and each fragment was cultured in the presence of antigen. The culture medium was changed at regular intervals, and the affinity of the antibodies was determined in those fragments which were producing antibody. The average affinity of the antibody from all the antibody-producing fragments was determined as well as the affinities of individual fragments.

As seen in Figure 6, some fragments produced antibody of high affinity and some fragments produced antibody of low affinity. This means that a cell-producing antibody of a given affinity lodged at that part of the spleen and began to proliferate in response to antigen. The antibody produced is the product of the progeny of that cell. This shows that antibody produced is clonal and the change in affinity is due to expansion of clones producing higher-affinity antibody having a proliferation advantage.

Antigen Selection Hypothesis

A unified theory to explain the change in affinity of the antibody produced has been proposed by Siskind and Benacerraf. Known as the ANTIGEN SELECTION HYPOTHESIS, this theory assumes that the binding properties of the antibody molecule which a cell synthesizes are a reflection of the binding properties of the membrane-associated recep-

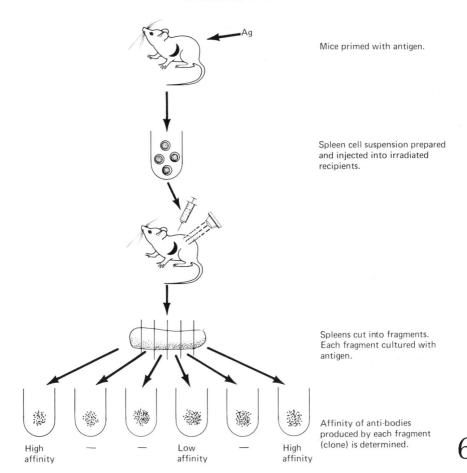

Mice primed with antigen.

Spleen cell suspension prepared and injected into irradiated recipients.

Spleens cut into fragments. Each fragment cultured with antigen.

Affinity of anti-bodies produced by each fragment (clone) is determined.

High affinity — — Low affinity — High affinity

6

Clonal nature of affinity of antibody-forming cells. [From Klinman (1969). *Immunochemistry,* **6, 757.]**

tor molecules of that cell. A cell which synthesizes high-affinity antibody would have high-affinity receptors, and a cell with low-affinity receptors would synthesize low-affinity antibody. This being the case, according to the theory there is competition among B-cells for the available antigen and, as in any evolutionary selective system, the "fittest" are selected. "Fittest" in this sense means having highest-affinity receptors. Selection here means that the cell which has the highest-affinity receptor also has the highest probability of reacting with antigen and of being induced to proliferate so that its progeny occupy a greater proportion of the population of antibody-forming cells than the unselected cell population. A given antigen will react specifically with those cells which have specific receptors, but of those cells with the proper specificity receptors, those with the highest affinity will have a greater chance of reacting with the antigen. These high-affinity cells will be induced to proliferate in preference to the cells with low-affinity receptors. By increasing their numbers more rapidly than other cells, high-affinity cells soon become the dominant members of the population, and the antibody which they synthesize soon occupies a greater proportion of the serum antibody molecules. As this selection of high-affinity cells occurs, a change in affinity is observed in the serum antibody. The change in affinity is not seen when high doses of antigen are used for immunization because there is sufficient antigen in the system that there is no competition for sites between high- and low-affinity cells, and cells with all affinities are stimulated at the same rate.

SUMMARY

1. Antigen induces proliferation of both helper and effector cells in antibody production and probably in cell-mediated responses.
2. The proliferation is specifically induced in those cells expressing antigen receptors for the specific antigen.
3. During the course of an antibody response there is a change in both the class and the affinity of the antibody produced. This is called the maturation of the antibody response.
4. The antibody produced in the early part of the primary antibody response is IgM. Late in the primary and throughout the secondary response IgG is produced. IgM is mercaptoethanol-sensitive, and IgG is mercaptoethanol-resistant.
5. It is not clear if a single effector cell switches from IgM to IgG production or if there are separate precursors for each class of Ig produced.
6. The affinity of the antibody produced changes during the secondary response. As the response progresses, the affinity increases.
7. The increase in affinity is thought to be due to the selection of effector cells expressing receptors of high affinity. This idea is strengthened by the fact that the affinity is clonally expressed. Clones of effector cells which produce higher-affinity antibody have a growth advantage over those expressing lower-affinity antibody.

READINGS

REVIEWS

Makinodan, T., and Albright, J. F. (1967). Proliferative and differentiative manifestations of cellular immune potential, *Prog. Allergy,* **10,** 1.

Uhr, J. W., and Finkelstein, M. S. (1967). The kinetics of antibody formation, *Prog. Allergy,* **10,** 37.
(These two reviews cover the problems of proliferation and maturation from an *in vivo* viewpoint.)
Dutton, R. W., and Mishell, R. I. (1967). Cellular events in the immune response. The *in vitro* response of normal spleen cells to erythrocyte antigens, *Cold Spring Harbor Symposium on Quant. Biol.* **32,** 407. (One of the first approaches to the problems of proliferation using *in vitro* methods.)
Siskind, G. W., and Benacerraf, B. (1969). Cell selection by antigen in the immune response, *Adv. Immunol.* **10,** 1. (A review of changing affinity with the elaboration of a selection model.)

18

REGULATOR T-CELLS

OVERVIEW

Some T-cells function as helper cells, other as effector cells. Another T-cell function, to act as suppressor or regulator, is thought to be of central importance in the immune response. In this chapter we will define several suppressor T-cell systems, both antigen specific and nonspecific, and show that a unique class of T-cells carries out this function.

SUPPRESSOR T-CELLS

One of the first intentional demonstrations of the suppressive role of the T-cell was the work of Richard Gershon. In a typical experiment, groups of adult mice were thymectomized, lethally irradiated, and reconstituted with syngeneic bone marrow. One group was then injected with thymus cells and the other was not. Both groups of mice were then given repeated doses of high concentrations of SRBC in an attempt to induce tolerance to the SRBC. After several weeks of this treatment, both groups received an injection of thymus cells as a source of helper cells and a challenge dose of SRBC. The anti-SRBC responses of both groups were measured, and it was found that the groups which had received thymus cells at the time of bone marrow reconstitution did not produce anti-SRBC antibody. This apparently anomalous result led to one of the most insightful interpretations of data in recent immunology. From this experiment and others like it

Gershon argued that the presence of the thymus cells during the course of injections with SRBC prevented the generation of an antibody response. This interpretation met with almost universal resistance. However, the idea of suppressor T-cells is now so universally accepted in cellular immunology that there is scarcely a phenomenon which is not explained by someone as being due to suppressor T-cells.

The role of the suppressor T-cell as regulator cell is inferred from the wide variety of situations in which suppression occurs in the immune response.

An example of a possible regulatory role of the T-cell comes from experiments in which mice were immunized with the thymus-independent antigen pneumococcus polysaccharide. If the mice were treated with *antilymphocyte serum* (ALS), a treatment which preferentially inactivates T-cells in the animal, a greater response to the pneumococcus polysaccharide was obtained than in untreated animals. This surprising result is best explained by postulating that the ALS removed a suppressor T-cell, thus allowing the mice to make a higher response to the antigen. In this case the regulatory role of the T-cell is to put a limit on the amount of anti-pneumococcus polysaccharide antibody which is produced. A somewhat similar finding occurs with lipopolysaccharide, another thymus-independent antigen.

Nonspecific Suppressor T-Cells Induced by ConA

In the course of examining the role of the T-cell mitogen ConA on *in vitro* antibody responses, Rich and Pierce noted that antibody responses were depressed when submitogenic doses of ConA were added to the cultures. To test the possibility that suppressor cells could be involved, they carried out what is now the standard experiment to check for suppression of antibody responses. The experiment is diagrammed in Figure 1. ConA was added to cultures of spleen cells. After 48 hr these cultures were washed and the cells added to a fresh culture of normal spleen cells. The antigen, SRBC, was added, and the cultures and controls were assayed at appropriate times for anti-SRBC plaque-forming cells (pfc). In this kind of experiment if a suppressor cell is present in the ConA-treated cultures, the normal cultures will not produce antibody; i.e., they will be suppressed. As seen in Figure 2, the culture of normal cells which had the added ConA-treated cells gave few pfc, meaning that the ConA-treated cells were preventing the normal cells from responding. If the ConA-treated culture was treated with anti-θ either before or after ConA was added, the suppressive activity was abolished. This showed that the cell responsible for the suppression was a T-cell.

A cell-free supernatant factor can be isolated from the ConA-

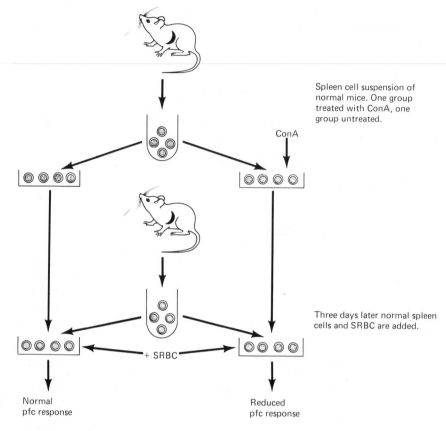

Spleen cell suspension of normal mice. One group treated with ConA, one group untreated.

ConA

Three days later normal spleen cells and SRBC are added.

+ SRBC

Normal pfc response

Reduced pfc response

1

Induction of suppressor T-cells with ConA. [After Rich and Pierce (1970). *J. Exp. Med.* 137, 205.]

treated cells which will carry out suppression in the absence of the cells. This soluble factor is a protein which does not react with antigen and is neither Ig nor H-2 in nature.

It is clear that the ConA-induced suppressor T-cell is nonspecific. This could mean that there are *nonspecific* suppressor cells which are activated by ConA or that there are a small number of naturally occurring suppressor cells which are antigen specific and that the ConA stimulation causes all these clones to be expanded.

Antigen-Specific Suppressor T-Cells

An example of antigen-specific suppressor cells is to be found in the experiments of Tada and his co-workers. In these experiments

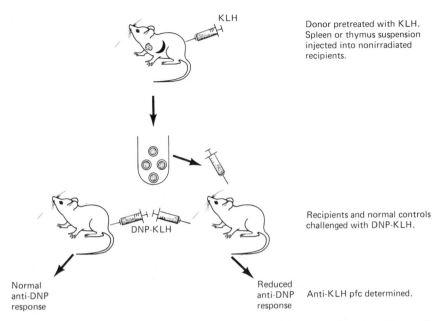

KLH

Donor pretreated with KLH.
Spleen or thymus suspension
injected into nonirradiated
recipients.

DNP-KLH

Recipients and normal controls
challenged with DNP-KLH.

Normal
anti-DNP
response

Reduced
anti-DNP
response

Anti-KLH pfc determined.

2

**Generation of antigen-specific suppressor T-cells. [After Tada *et al.*
(1974). *J. Exp. Med.* 140, 239.]**

which are diagrammed in Figure 2, mice are primed with a high dose
of carrier, and the thymocytes or spleens of these mice are then
transferred to syngeneic unirradiated recipients which are challenged
with hapten and carrier. The response of the recipients to the hapten
is suppressed under these conditions.

If the primed cells are treated with anti-θ and complement before
transfer to the nonirradiated recipients, the suppression is abolished.
This argues that a T-cell in the primed population is acting as a
suppressor cell. Furthermore, if the donors are pretreated with carrier A and the recipient mice are challenged with the hapten on
carrier B, there is no suppression. This indicates that the suppression
is *antigen specific*.

In the chapters on helper-effector interactions we saw that one
possible mode of action between B-cells and T-cells for generating
antibody responses was the antigen-induced elaboration of soluble
products which are liberated by specific interaction of antigen and
T-cell. Once liberated, some of these factors acted nonspecifically on
other cells. Others, however, acted only on specific cells. To begin to
approach this question in this suppressor system, mice were primed

with carrier A, and the thymocytes transferred to nonirradiated recipients which were then challenged with hapten conjugated to carrier B plus free carrier A. The reasoning here was that if antigen reacted with the suppressor cells and a nonspecific factor was elaborated, the reaction of antigen A and cells primed to A should be sufficient to cause the factor to be released if a soluble factor is operating in this sytem. If there is a factor and if, once released, it acts nonspecifically, then the response of the mice to the hapten conjugated to carrier B should be suppressed. When this experiment was carried out, the response to hapten on carrier B was found *not* to be suppressed. This argued that the specific interaction of antigen and cell does not cause release of a soluble factor which acts nonspecifically.

Even though specific antigen interaction does not cause release *in vivo* of a soluble factor which acts nonspecifically, a factor can be obtained from the suppressor cells *in vitro*. This factor is obtained by disrupting the primed population of T-cells by sonication. When injected into the recipient mice, the sonicated product causes antigen-specific suppression. The molecule is a protein with molecular weight of 35,000 to 60,000 daltons.

The suppressor molecule obtained in this way is not removed on an anti-Ig column, but an anti-H-2 column removes the activity. When anti-I region antisera were bound to the column, it was found that the factor was removed more efficiently by anti-I region specificities (Ia) than by anti-K or D specificities. Furthermore, the factor reacts with antigen. The similarity between this factor and the helper factor of Taussig and Munro (Chapter 9) is very striking. Both are T-cell products which have antigen-binding capacity but are Ia rather than Ig.

Another feature of this factor is the characteristic that it can be absorbed onto the surface of the cells which are suppressed. Only θ-positive cells bind the factor, indicating that it may act on a helper T-cell. But of most interest is the fact that cells from mice of B10 background cannot be suppressed by this factor because they lack an *acceptor* for it on their cell surface. Even though B10 congenics cannot be suppressed by the factor, they are able to produce it. A-strain mice, in contrast, cannot produce the factor but have a receptor for it. An F_1 of (B10.A × A), a nonacceptor and a nonproducer, are able both to produce and accept the factor. We must of course bear in mind that the suppression *in vivo* is not by a soluble product and that the suppressor factor is obtained only by sonication of the cells. This argues that while the suppressor molecule may be of physiological importance, it may function by membrane interaction between the acceptor and suppressor molecules. This would suggest that cell contact might be needed for suppression to occur in nature. In the next two suppressor systems to be discussed, we will see that cell contact is required for at least these two forms of suppression by T-cells.

Suppression by Spontaneous T-Cell Leukemias

It has been known for some time that mice bearing tumors often have impaired immune responses. This is true of AKR mice, which is a high leukemia strain. AKR mice develop a spontaneous thymic leukemia at about 6 months of age, and once leukemic are unable to generate immune responses. The leukemic cells, which are malignant T-cells, have been shown to be acting as suppressor cells by mixing them with normal AKR cells.

Two facts about the nature of these suppressor cells which may have bearing on suppressor T-cells in general have emerged from the work of Roman and Golub. They were able to show that the suppression by AKR leukemias is not mediated by soluble factors but that *cell contact* is probably involved. This was done by showing that supernatant fluids of cultures of leukemic cells, when added to normal cultures, did not suppress them. A more rigorous experiment was one in which the normal and leukemic cells were grown in chambers which were separated by a cell-impermeable but fluid-permeable membrane. Even under conditions in which the culture fluids of the two cell types were constantly being exchanged, there was no suppression of normal cells.

The second point to emerge from the study of AKR suppressor cells has been that most, but not all, spontaneous tumors will suppress only AKR and not allogeneic strains (Figure 3). The reason for this genetic restriction has been explained by the fact that allogeneic interaction results in the production of a factor which overcomes suppression. Those leukemic cells which suppress only AKR and in which the suppression is overcome by allogeneic cells and supernates are called RESTRICTED SUPPRESSOR CELLS. Those which suppress all strains are termed NONRESTRICTED SUPPRESSOR CELLS. The nonrestricted suppressors are not affected by allogeneic cells and supernatants. The reason for the restricted and nonrestricted nature of the suppression is not known, but the fact that contact is needed shows that membrane-associated molecules may be very important.

Suppressor T-Cells in Neonatal Mice

Newborn animals in general have impaired immune capacities (Chapter 12). We now think that this is due in part at least to the

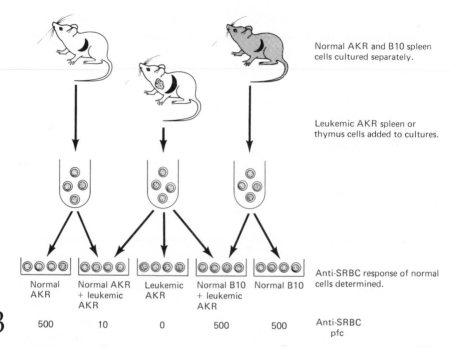

					Normal AKR and B10 spleen cells cultured separately.
					Leukemic AKR spleen or thymus cells added to cultures.
Normal AKR	Normal AKR + leukemic AKR	Leukemic AKR	Normal B10 + leukemic AKR	Normal B10	Anti-SRBC response of normal cells determined.
500	10	0	500	500	Anti-SRBC pfc

3

Leukemic AKR suppressor cells suppress normal responses of AKR but not allogeneic cells. [After Roman and Golub (1976). *J. Exp. Med.* 143, 482.]

presence of suppressor T-cells in the thymus and spleens of newborn mice. This was first demonstrated by Johnson and Mosier in experiments in which cells from 1-week old mice were shown to be able to make normal responses to thymus-independent antigens but not to thymus-dependent responses. When the young cells were mixed with adult cells, the responses of the adult cells to a thymus-dependent antigen were suppressed. The suppression was carried out by a T-cell which was present from birth to several weeks of age, depending on the strain of mouse.

When the neonatal suppressor cell was examined in more detail by Durdik and Golub, the suppression was found not to be exerted by a soluble factor but rather by cell contact. This makes the neonatal suppressor cell very similar to the leukemic suppressor cell.

Allotype Suppression

Another system in which suppressor T-cells play a role is ALLOTYPE SUPPRESSION. In this system, when a neonatal animal is exposed to antibody against its own immunoglobulin, the production of these immunoglobulins is suppressed.[1] An animal that is heterozygous for allotypes *a* and *b* has the genes for immunoglobulin allotypes *a* and *b* and will have some Ig molecules which are allotype *a* and some which are allotype *b* (see Chapter 13 for a review of allotypes). But if anti-*a* antibody has been injected into the animal when it was a newborn, then only allotype *b* will be synthesized by the adult; i.e., the cells producing anti-*a* cease their production. In the experiments of Mage and Dray rabbits heterozygous for allotypes b_4b_5 were injected at birth with anti-b_4. These animals had no b_4 Ig molecules in their serum even a year after treatment, while noninjected littermates had normal levels.

In the mouse a similar phenomenon occurs, but except for one strain combination, the suppression is short-term. In experiments of the Herzenbergs, in normal mice the level of Ig in the serum reaches maximum values at approximately 8 weeks after birth, while in heterozygous progeny whose mothers were immunized to the paternal allotype, the level of the suppressed allotype reaches adult values at approximately 15 weeks. The strain combination which shows *chronic allotype suppression* is (SJL × BALB/c)F_1. BALB/c have Iga allotype molecules, and SJL have Igb allotypes. If BALB/c females are immunized to Igb and mated to SJL males, some of the offspring have severely depressed Igb levels. In the 50 percent of the offspring which are suppressed, the suppression lasts for up to 6 months of age. It may be important to note that a variety of other strains, when mated to immune BALB/c females do not show this chronic suppression, and only half of the (SJL × BALB/c) mice show it. SJL is known to have anomalies in its immune system, and chronic allotype suppression in this strain combination may be a reflection of these anomalies.

Whatever the significance of this phenomenon it can be shown that chronic allotype suppression may be mediated by suppressor T-cells. This is shown by the following experiment. Irradiated BALB/c mice repopulated with normal (BALB × SJL)F_1 spleen cells produce both Iga and Igb, but repopulation with suppressed (BALB × SJL)F_1 spleen cells result in only Iga production. Mixtures of spleen cells from chronically suppressed (SJL × BALB)F_1 and normal (SJL × BALB)F_1, when injected into irradiated BALB recipients, results in

---

[1]Ig molecules of only one parental allotype are secreted by individual cells in an F animal. This phenomenon is called ALLELIC EXCLUSION. In allelic exclusion, some lymphocytes of a heterozygous F_1 produce Ig molecules of one parental type and some produce molecules of the other even though the genes for both are present. No cells produce both types of molecules.

only Iga production, which shows that Igb production by the recipients is suppressed. It appears that the normal (SJL × BALB)F$_1$ cells are prevented from producing Igb by the Igb-suppressed spleens. When the suppressed spleens are treated with anti-θ before transfer, the suppressive activity is abolished. This is a strong argument for suppressor T-cells being important in allotype suppression.

Suppressor Cells in Human Immunodeficiency Disease

There are a series of immune deficiency diseases in man. In one of these, common variable hypogammaglobulinemia (CVH), a possible suppressor lymphocyte has been identified. When the circulating lymphocytes of normal humans are incubated with the B-cell mitogen pokeweek (Chapter 5), there is increased production of immunoglobulin by the B-cells. Patients with CVH do not show this increase in immunoglobulin after pokeweed mitogen stimulation. When mixtures of normal and CVH lymphocytes are incubated with pokeweed mitogen, the normal cells are prevented from synthesizing immunoglobulin. There is some evidence that the lymphocyte which is preventing the synthesis is a T-cell. Thus this form of immunodeficiency in man may be the result of suppressor T-cells.

Surface Antigens on Suppressor Cells

We know from the material in Section II that helper cells in both antibody and cell-mediated reactions are θ positive and express Ly 1. The effector cells in the CML response are θ positive and express Ly 2, 3. The natural question was to determine the Ly profile of the suppressor T-cell. To test their surface antigens, both nonspecific (ConA) and specific suppressors (to SRBC) were generated and treated with anti-Ly 1 or anti-Ly 2 and 3 to determine if the suppressor cell is Ly 1 or Ly 2, 3 positive. It was found that in both cases the suppressor T-cell is Ly 2, 3 positive and Ly 1 negative. This means that the suppressor T-cell has the same Ly profile as the cytotoxic cell. It immediately becomes evident that the suppressor T-cell could be a form of cytotoxic effector cell directed against helper cells. This becomes even more plausible when one considers that recognition of altered self through H-2 molecules has recently been shown to exist and to be of potential importance. An experiment which can determine if the Ly 2, 3 suppressor T-cell and cytotoxic effector cells are different cells becomes very important. Such an experiment has now been carried out by at least two groups, and the results point clearly to the fact that the suppressor and cytotoxic cells are *different* cells.

The experiment consisted of generating both suppressor cells and cytotoxic cells and treating them with anti-θ, anti-Ly, or anti-Ia antisera plus complement. As expected (Table 1), both suppressor and cytotoxic cells were killed by anti-θ and complement. Treatment with anti-Ly 1 had no effect on either, but treatment with anti-Ly 2, 3 removed both activities. When anti-Ia and complement were used, it was found that cytotoxic T-cells were Ia negative but that suppressor T-cells were Ia positive. Thus the two functional cell types have different surface antigens, which argues that they are different cell populations.

Very recently both allotype suppression and antigen specific suppression have been found to be associated with a new subregion of the I region of H-2. This region, termed I-J, maps between IB and IC.

LYMPHOKINES

T-cells produce substances which alter the physiology of other cells. These substances are called LYMPHOKINES. Some immunologists argue that the production of lymphokines correlates well with other cell-mediated responses (DTH, for example). If these substances do have physiological function, it is in the tissue damage seen in cell-mediated responses.

Migration-Inhibiting Factor

If peritoneal exudate cells of a mouse are cultured in a capillary tube, macrophages migrate from the end of the tube, forming a fan of cells. If the cells are from a sensitized mouse and the antigen to which the mouse is sensitized is added to the culture, the macrophages are inhibited from migrating from the tube. The inhibition of migration

TABLE 1.   TREATMENT OF SUPPRESSOR AND CYTOTOXIC T-CELLS WITH ALLOANTISERA TO DETERMINE IF THEY ARE SEPARATE CELL POPULATIONS.

Treatment with	Effect on function	
	Suppressor	Cytotoxic
Anti-θ + C	Abolished	Abolished
Anti-Ly 1 + C	No effect	No effect
Anti-Ly 2, 3 + C	Abolished	Abolished
Anti-Ia + C	Abolished	No effect

Data from Janchinski et al. (1976). J. Exp. Med. **143,** 1382; Cantor et al. (1976). J. Exp. Med. **143,** 1391; Huber et al. (1976). J. Exp. Med. **143,** 1534.

is antigen specific since adding an antigen other than the one used for sensitization to the culture does not inhibit migration.

The cell responsible for the prevention of macrophage migration is a T-cell. Treatment of the peritoneal exudates with anti-θ and complement abolishes the ability to inhibit migration. The sensitized T-cell reacts with antigen and liberates a soluble product called MACROPHAGE INHIBITING FACTOR (MIF). This factor is a nonimmunoglobulin with a molecular weight of between 35,000 and 55,000 daltons. MIF reacts with macrophages and prevents their migration. Whatever the physiological role, if any, of MIF, it is a very good assay for sensitized T-cells. MACROPHAGE AGGREGATION FACTOR (MAF) is another factor which sensitized T-cells liberate after reaction with antigen. It causes macrophages to aggregate.

Lymphotoxin

Lymphocytes stimulated with mitogens or after infection with some virus liberate a factor into the culture supernatants which is toxic for other lymphocytes. Termed LYMPHOTOXIN (LT), this material is assayed by measuring the decrease in viable target cells after treatment.

Chemotactic Factor

The DTH lesion in an animal has accumulated macrophages. A factor, probably liberated by T-cells, has been found in culture which is chemotactic for macrophages.

SUMMARY

1. A subset of T-cells can function as cells which suppress the immune response. These are called suppressor T-cells.
2. Suppressor T-cells can be induced by treating spleen populations with low doses of ConA. These are nonspecific suppressor T-cells. Antigen-specific suppressor T-cells can be generated by treating animals with high doses of carrier; after transfer to unirradiated recipients the anti-hapten response of the host to hapten conjugated to the carrier is suppressed.
3. ConA-induced suppressor T-cells elaborate a soluble factor which is suppressive. A factor which carries out suppression can be isolated from antigen-specific suppressor cells.
4. Nonspecific suppressor T-cells which act by cell contact are found in spontaneous AKR leukemia and normal neonatal mice.
5. Suppressor T-cells express Ly 2, 3 on their surfaces but are distinguished from cytotoxic cells, which are also Ly 2, 3, by the fact that they are Ia positive, whereas cytotoxic cells are Ly negative. A new subregion of the I region, I-J, may be expressed exclusively on suppressor T-cells.

6. Lymphokines are soluble products of activated T-cells which alter the physiology of other cells. Their products may play a role in the tissue damage seen in some cell-mediated responses.

READINGS

REVIEWS

Gershon, R. K. (1974). T-cell control of antibody production, *Contemp. Top. Immunobiol.* **3**, 1. (A superb review of the evidence which led to the discovery of the suppressor T-cell.)

Bloom, B. R. (1971). *In vitro* approaches to the mechanism of cell-mediated immune reactions, *Adv. Immunol.* **13**, 101. (An old, but complete, review of lymphokines.)

ARTICLES

Rich, R. R., and Pierce, C. W. (1974). Biological expressions of lymphocyte activation. III. Suppression of plaque-forming cell responses *in vitro* by supernatant fluids from Concanavalian A-activated spleen cell cultures, *J. Immunol.* **112**, 1360. (Nonspecific suppression by mitogen-stimulated cells mediated by a soluble factor.)

Roman, J. R. and Golub, E. S. (1976). Leukemia in AKR mice. I. Effects of leukemic cells on antibody-forming potential of syngeneic and allogeneic normal cells, *J. Exp. Med.* **143**, 482. (Nonspecific suppression by leukemic cells mediated by cell contact.)

Takemori, T., and Tada, T. (1975). Properties of antigen-specific suppressive T-cell factor in the regulation of antibody response of the mouse. I. *In vivo* activity and immunochemical characterizations, *J. Exp. Med.* **142**, 1241.

Tada, T., Taniguchi, M., and David, C. S. (1976). Properties of the antigen-specific suppressive T-cell factor in the regulation of antibody response in the mouse. III. Special subregion assignment of the gene(s) that code for the suppressive T-cell factor in the H-2 histocompatability complex, *J. Exp. Med.* **144**, 713. (Antigen-specific suppression.)

19

GENETICS OF THE IMMUNE RESPONSE

OVERVIEW

Variability in the magnitude of immune responses of random-bred animals has been recognized as a fact of life by several generations of immunologists. Some of this variability has been known for a long time to have a genetic basis.

The widespread use of highly inbred strains of mice has tended to reduce the variability of responses since responses to any given antigen are more uniform within an inbred strain. However, part of the laboratory lore of the practicing immunologist is the fact that some inbred strains are better responders to certain antigens than are others.

In this chapter we will discuss in detail two systems of genetic control of the immune response. The first is the PLL gene in the guinea pig, and the second is the Ir-1 gene in the mouse. We will see that the genes controlling many immune responses are localized in the major histocompatability locus (H-2 and HLA). The function of these genes is probably connected in some manner with antigen recognition.

BREEDING OF HIGH- AND LOW-RESPONDING MICE

As an example of the genetic control over the magnitude of an antibody response, it is possible to select lines of good- and poor-responding animals from random-bred mice. If random-bred mice

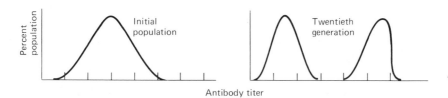

High- and low-responder mice to SRBC. Percent of population making antibody response of given magnitude. [After Biozzi (1971). *Prog. Immunol.* 1, 529.]

which make high responses to a certain antigen are mated with other random-bred mice which also make high responses, after a few generations lines of high-responding animals are obtained. An example of this is seen in the data in Figure 1. In this experiment random-bred mice were injected with SRBC, and the titer of anti-SRBC in the serum determined. Those individuals which produced high titers of anti-SRBC antibody were mated with mice which also made high responses. The selection procedure was repeated at each generation until a divergence in the two lines was seen. This kind of experiment shows that the ability to make high or low responses to an antigen is under some form of genetic control.

PLL GENE

Genetic Control of Anti-PLL Response

The pioneering work on the genetic control of the immune response was carried out by Benacerraf and his students and co-workers on the PLL gene of the guinea pig. When the hapten DNP was conjugated to the carrier poly-L-lysine (PLL), emulsified in Freund's complete adjuvant, and injected into randomly bred Hartley guinea pigs, it was found that 30 percent of the animals made immune responses to the DNP hapten and 70 percent did not. This shows that in a non-inbred population some animals respond to this antigen and others do not. To determine if the ability and inability to respond are under genetic control, responder guinea pigs were mated with other responders. It was found that 80 percent of the offspring of this cross were responders. Mating nonresponders with nonresponders resulted in 100 percent nonresponders.

Known:

Responder × responder = responder (80%) + nonresponder (20%)
Nonresponder × nonresponder = nonresponder (100%)

If the control of the response is due to a single gene, then the genotypes could be RR and Rr for the responders and rr for the nonresponders. To test this, one can mate heterozygous responders to nonresponders and determine the response of the offspring. A *homozygous responder* is an animal whose parents are both responders. A *heterozygous responder* is an animal which is a responder but who has one parent who is a nonresponder.

Homozygous responder: RR
Heterozygous responder: Rr
Nonresponder: rr

When the experiment was carried out, the proportion of responders and nonresponders was found to be what one would expect from a single dominant gene.

Predicted:

50% responders + 50% nonresponders

Rr × rr = 2 Rr + 2 rr

Obtained:

45.3% responders + 54.7% nonresponders

This finding is consistent with the control of the response to DNP-PLL being under a single dominant gene. The response is not sex linked, thus showing that the gene is autosomal.

Antibody and Cell-Mediated Responses to DNP-PLL

The responder animals made both antibody and cell-mediated responses (delayed-type hypersensitivity to antigen injected into the skin) to DNP-PLL. The nonresponder animals were nonresponders for both antibody and cell-mediated responses. It was then important to determine if the nonresponders were able to respond to the hapten DNP on another carrier. Both responders and nonresponders were found to make normal responses to DNP when it was conjugated to any other carrier. This showed that the genetic control was not for DNP. When guinea pigs were immunized to other haptens conjugated to PLL, it was found that responders produced both antibody and cell-mediated responses against any hapten on the PLL carrier. The nonresponders, however, were unable to produce either antibody or cell-mediated response to any hapten conjugated to PLL. Since the nonresponders were able to make normal responses to DNP or any hapten conjugated to carriers other than PLL, this indicated that the nonresponders were unable to respond to the PLL and the gene was controlling the response to PLL. The gene was thus named the *PLL gene*.

Failure to Recognize PLL

If the failure to respond to PLL is failure to recognize it, this lack of recognition should be circumvented in antibody formation by complexing DNP-PLL to another molecule and allowing the other molecule to act as carrier. To test this, DNP-PLL was electrostatically complexed to an acetylated form of BSA and injected into nonresponders. These nonresponders were able to make anti-DNP responses even though the DNP was conjugated to PLL because the PLL was complexed to the BSA. The nonresponders were using helper cells directed to the BSA in the anti-DNP response.

When the cell-mediated responses were examined in the DNP-PLL-BSA immunized animals, it was found that nonresponders failed to make cell-mediated responses to PLL. This shows that the nonresponders have effector cells for anti-DNP antibody and can use the BSA helper cells but they lack PLL helper cells and also lack PLL effector cells in cell-mediated responses. These findings are summarized in Table 1.

Further evidence that the defect in the nonresponders was due to lack of cells able to recognize the carrier molecule was obtained by making nonresponder animals specifically unresponsive to BSA by inducing a state of immunological tolerance to BSA (details in Chapter 20). A tolerant animal cannot respond to the specific antigen to which it is tolerant but can make normal responses to other antigens. When DNP-PLL-BSA was injected into BSA-tolerant nonresponders, they should not have been able to use the BSA as a carrier in making an anti-DNP response since BSA helper cells are nonfunctional in a BSA-tolerant animal. This is exactly the result that was obtained; the tolerant nonresponders failed to produce anti-DNP antibody to the DNP-PLL-BSA complex.

TABLE 1. RESPONSES OF NONRESPONDER GUINEA PIGS TO DNP-PLL AND DNP-PLL-BSA.

Nonresponder immunized with	Anti-DNP response	Delayed hypersensitivity to PLL
DNP-PLL	No	No
DNP-PLL-BSA	Yes	No

After Benacerraf et al. (1967). Cold Spring Harbor Symposium on Quantitative Biology, **32,** 569.

The conclusion which we can draw from this elegant series of experiments is that both the responder and nonresponder guinea pigs have the genetic information to produce antibody to the DNP (i.e., effector B-cells) but that *nonresponders fail to respond to the carrier*, showing that they lack helper T-cells. They also lack effector cells in cell-mediated responses, showing that the defect in nonresponder guinea pigs to PLL is at the level of T-cell recognition. These experiments are even more instructive in telling us about scientific insight since they were carried out before the clear delineation of helper and carrier functions of antigen and lymphocytes.

Similar studies have also been carried out in two inbred strains of guinea pigs, strain 2 and strain 13. Strain-2 guinea pigs are responders, and strain 13 are nonresponders. It will be seen in the next section that this is an example of the widespread association of immune response genes with major histocompatability loci. The mouse is the animal of choice to study histocompatability-associated phenomena, and the next section deals with one such MHC-associated immune response gene (Ir-1) in detail.

Ir-1 GENE

Studies with Polypeptide Antigens

The study of the genetics of the immune response in mice has been carried out using copolymers of amino acids. When *random copolymers* of glutamic acid, alanine, and tyrosine (GAT) or glutamic acid, lysine, and alanine (GLA) were injected into various strains of mice, it was found that some strains made good antibody responses while others were poor responders. By doing the appropriate crosses and backcrosses, it was determined that responsiveness was probably due to a single, dominant gene.

Other extensively used synthetic polypeptide antigens employed in studying the genetics of the immune response are *branched, multichained amino acid copolymers*. These copolymers consist of a polylysine backbone with side chains of poly-DL-alanine and various amino acids attached to the alanine side chains. A schematic diagram of one of the most commonly used branched-chain copolymers, tyrosine-glutamic-alanine-lysine (TGAL), is shown in Figure 2. By using histidine or phenylalanine as one of the amino acids, HGAL or PGAL is obtained.

Discovery of Ir-1 Gene

McDevitt and his co-workers showed that when TGAL is emulsified in Freund's complete adjuvant and injected into CBA and

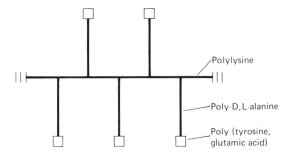

A schematic diagram of the structural pattern of (T,G)–A–L. [From H. O. McDevitt and M. Sela (1965). *J. Exp. Med.* **122**, 517.]

C57BL/6 mice, a clear difference in the amount of antibody produced by each strain can be seen (Figure 3). In this case the CBA mice make low responses, and the C57BL/6 make high responses. The (CBA × C57BL)F$_1$ make responses intermediate between the two parental types.

Since the PLL response and the response to GAT are under single gene control, it would be predicted that the response to TGAL might be under similar control. To test this, the responses of the high-responding strain (C57BL/6), the low-responding strain (CBA), the F$_1$, and the F$_1$ backcrossed to each parental strain were tested.

If control is by a single gene, then the parental high responders are HH and the parental low responders are LL. A cross should give:

HH × LL = HL

As seen in Figure 3, this is what was found experimentally. The F$_1$ made a response intermediate between the two parental responses.

Under single gene control a backcross of the F$_1$ to high responding parent should give:

HL × HH = HH + HL

This was obtained (Figure 3); the F$_1$ × C57BL/6 cross gives predominantly high responders. Similarly, a backcross of the F$_1$ to the low responder should give low and intermediate responders.

All this is consistent with the response to TGAL being under single gene control. The responses to HGAL and PGAL were also found to be controlled by this gene, which was named immune response-1 (Ir-1).

Association of Ir Gene with H-2

Many strains of mice were screened to determine if they were high or low responders to TGAL and other antigens. A very striking

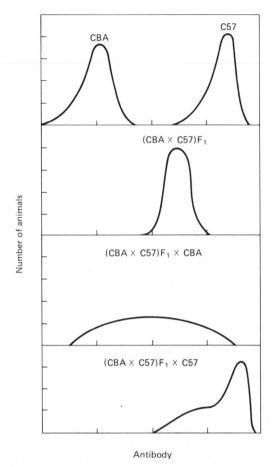

3

Antibody responses of CBA, C57, and crosses to TGAL. [After H. O. McDevitt and M. Sela (1965). *J. Exp. Med.* 122, 517.]

picture soon began to emerge; the ability to be a high responder to a given antigen was associated with certain H-2 haplotypes. Different antigens showed different patterns of high and low responders, but within the haplotype the animals were consistent in their responses.

To prove that the control over responsiveness to TGAL is actually exerted by genes within the H-2 complex, congenic and recombinant mice were used. It will be recalled from Chapter 6 that these mice have identical background genes but different H-2 genes. For example, C3H mice which are H-2^k are low responders to TGAL, but C57BL/6 which is H-2^b is a high responder. The congenic strain

C3H.SW, having the same background genes as C3H but having H-2 genes which are H-2^b, is a high responder to TGAL. Thus when background genes are identical, it is the H-2 haplotype which determines if the animals will be high or low responders. Another example is strain B10 which is a high responder to TGAL and is H-2^b. The congenic strain B10.BR has identical background genes to B10 but has the H-2^k haplotype. These H-2^k mice are low responders, showing again that the differences in the H-2 haplotype are crucial for control of the antibody response to TGAL.

The next problem was *to localize the position of the gene* responsible for this control within the H-2 complex. This was done using H-2 recombinant mice (Chapter 6). The recombinants which had known differences in H-2 genes were immunized, and the correlation of each of the known regions of the H-2 complex with the immune response was noted. Previously we have discussed H-2 haplotypes in terms of six regions (for example, kkkkkk). At the time these studies were carried out, only the K, S, and D regions were known. By use of the recombinant mice the gene controlling the response to TGAL was localized between K and S, forming a new region. The new region was termed the I region, for immune response, and the H-2 map then had four regions, K, I, S, and D. At least three subregions of I have since been discovered, and so we know that the H-2 map is K, IA, IB, IC, S, and D.

Since the realization in the early 1960s that the genetic control of the immune response to TGAL was in the H-2 complex, the responses to a vast number of antigens have been tested to determine if they are under genetic control. The responses to at least 15 antigens have been shown to be controlled by genes in the H-2 region. The process of localizing the genes within the subregions continues at a rapid pace.

Two-Gene Control

Recent evidence shows that the responses to TGAL, GLT, and GLφ (GL phenylalanine) are under the control of two genes in the I region of the H-2 complex. This conclusion comes from data seen in Table 2. If there were one-gene control, as thought from the original data, then the mating of nonresponders with nonresponders would always lead to nonresponders. The fact that there are two genes both localized within the H-2 complex is suggested by the finding that a cross between low responders to TGAL, B10.BR, and B10.M, leads to a high responder. Similarly, with GLφ as antigen, A and B10 are both low responders, yet the F_1 gives a high responder. It has been postulated that these two genes act in a cis-trans manner.

TABLE 2. EVIDENCE FOR TWO-GENE CONTROL OF THE RESPONSE TO SOME ANTIGENS.

Antigen	Strain	H-2	Response
TGAL	B10.BR	k	Low
	I.SE	d	Low
	B10.M	f	Low
	(B10.BR × I.SE)F$_1$		High
	(B10.BR × B10.M)F$_1$		High
GLϕ	A	a	Low
	B10	b	Low
	(A × B10)F$_1$		High
	(A × B10.A)F$_1$		Low

Data on TGAL from Munro and Taussig (1975). *Nature* **256,** 103; data on GLϕ from Dorf *et al.* (1975). *J. Exp. Med.* **141,** 1457.

Site of Action

Up to this point we have shown that responsiveness to a variety of antigens is controlled by genes in the I region of the H-2 complex. It is now important to look at the evidence for the cellular site at which the gene is expressed and if possible to determine the mode of action.

To determine if the defect in the nonresponders was expressed in the lymphocytes associated with the immune response or if there was some kind of environmental factor in the nonresponders which prevents cells from responding, spleen cells from responder F$_1$ mice were injected into lethally irradiated nonresponder parental mice. The recipients were challenged with TGAL and the antibody titers determined. The responder cells were able to produce anti-TGAL antibody in the nonresponder hosts. This shows that the environment of the nonresponder animal is able to support an immune response and strongly suggests that the defect in the nonresponder is at the cellular level.

It was already known from work on the PLL gene in guinea pigs that the defect in PLL low responders was at the level of recognition and that functional effector cells for antibody formation could be demonstrated by immunizing low responders with antigen complexed to BSA. The same experiment was carried out in nonresponder mice in the TGAL system. When low responders were immunized with TGAL complexed to BSA, they were converted to high responders.

This shows that functional B-cells are present in the nonresponders and seems to point to a T-cell defect.

Insight into a possible T-cell defect in nonresponder mice is found in the observation that both responder and nonresponder mice make the same amount of anti-TGAL in response to primary injection of TGAL in saline (rather than adjuvant). When a second injection is given, however, only responder mice make a secondary response. Furthermore, the antibody made by both responder and nonresponder mice in the primary response is IgM (mercaptoethanol-sensitive), but the antibody made in the secondary is IgG (mercaptoethanol-resistant). After thymectomy, however, responder mice function like nonresponders; i.e., they make only 19s and not 7s anti-TGAL. This was shown in experiments using C3H.SW responders and comparing the responses of thymectomized and intact animals. After thymectomy C3H.SW responder mice produce only 19s anti-TGAL antibody and no 7s; i.e., they function like C3H nonresponder mice.

This data has been used to argue that the defect in nonresponders is at the T-cell and also that one function of the T-cell may be to bring about the switch from IgM to IgG (see Chapter 17) since only responders can make a 7s response.

Evidence for Impaired B- and T-Cell Function

The data cited above points to a T-cell defect, but the picture is far from complete as can be seen from the following data. In Chapter 9 we saw that factors from T-cells could substitute for T-cells in carrying out helper function in B:T cooperation. One of the T-cell factors has antigen specificity and is made up of an H-2 product. This factor was obtained from responder mice and was injected along with bone marrow cells from either responder or nonresponder mice into irradiated mice which were challenged with TGAL. In this way it was hoped to determine if the defect in the nonresponder was at the level of inability to produce the factor or inability to respond to it. Apparently conflicting results have come out of these experiments. When the strains of mice are C3H.SW as responders and C3H as nonresponders, the defect seems to be a B-cell defect; i.e., the bone marrow of nonresponders does not interact with factor from responders. In this case the responder and nonresponder T-cells both produce a factor which allows responder B-cells to produce anti-TGAL antibody, but the nonresponder B-cells do not respond to the T-cell factor from either set of T-cells. However, when the nonresponder strain is SJL, the defect appears to be in both B-cells and T-cells. In this case, factor from responder T-cells allows responder B-cells to produce antibody, but nonresponder B-cells do not react. Similarly, the SJL nonresponder T-cells are deficient in generating a T-cell factor to react with responder B-cells.

This conflict in data can now perhaps be best explained by the two-gene control. One gene may be expressed in B-cells and one gene may be expressed in T-cells in different strains. This notion is currently being tested in several laboratories.

Evidence for Suppressor T-Cells

A variation of the T-cell defect in some cases of genetic nonresponsiveness is that the T-cell is acting as a *suppressor cell* (see Chapter 18). The response to the polypeptide GAT is under H-2-linked genetic control, and just as in the cases of DNP-PLL and TGAL, the nonresponder mice make antibody when the antigen is electrostatically conjugated to BSA. By this criterion nonresponders to GAT have functional B-cells. Nonresponder mice, however, fail to become converted to respond by BSA-GAT if they first receive an injection of GAT. In other words, pretreatment with the unconjugated antigen prevents the mice from responding to antigen conjugated to BSA. This could be a form of immunological tolerance (Chapter 20), or it could be due to the presence of *suppressor T-cells*.

To test the alternative hypotheses, the experiment in Figure 4 was carried out. Spleen cells from GAT-treated nonresponder mice were mixed with cells from untreated nonresponders in a Mishell-Dutton *in vitro* system and challenged with GAT-BSA. If pretreatment with GAT induces the production of suppressor cells in the nonresponders, then they should prevent normal nonpretreated nonresponder cells from responding to GAT-BSA. This is the result obtained in the experiment. It was found that the untreated cells were unable to respond to GAT-BSA; i.e., they were suppressed when co-cultured with pretreated cells. This suppression could be reversed if the GAT-treated cells were first treated with anti-θ serum to eliminate T-cells. When this is done, the suppression is removed and the untreated group responds to GAT-BSA. This argues that the cell responsible for suppression is a θ-positive cell, i.e., a T-cell. Hence in this system it appears that the suppressor T-cell may play a role in genetic control of unresponsiveness.

IMMUNE RESPONSE GENES IN MAN

In man there is a clear association between HLA type and certain diseases. A few examples are given in Table 3. Since the HLA of man is the analogue of H-2 in the mouse, the fact that resistance or

Normal mice or GAT-pretreated mice.

Spleen cells either plated alone or mixed together. One mixed group is treated with anti-θ + C.

Anti-θ + C

Normal	Normal + GAT pre-treated	Normal + GAT pretreated anti-θ treated	GAT pretreated
1,250	350	1,000	125

Anti-GAT response determined.

4

Presence of a suppressor T-cell in GAT-pretreated spleen populations. [After Benacerraf, Kapp, and Pierce, in Katz and Benacerraf (1974). *Immunological Tolerance*, 507.]

TABLE 3. ASSOCIATIONS BETWEEN HLA TYPE AND DISEASE

Disease	*Associated HLA Antigen*
Hodgkin's disease	HLA5
Chronic myelogenous leukemia	HLA3, HLA12
Acute lymphocytic leukemia	HLA2, HLA12, HLA1
Lymphosarcoma	HLA12
Systemic lupus erythematosus	HLA8, W15
Chronic glomerulonephritis	HLA2
Gluten-sensitive enteropathy	HLA8
Dermatitis herpetiformis	HLA8
Psoriasis	HLA13, HLA17
Ankylosing spondylitis	HLAW27

From Green (1974). *Immunogenetics*, **1,** 4.

susceptibility to disease is associated with HLA leads naturally to analogy of the I region. It is only natural that most associations are with susceptibility to disease since it is through analysis of diseased patients with the HLA type that the association is made. Extended family studies must be performed to localize the gene(s) associated with disease susceptibility within the H-2 complex.

SUMMARY

1. The ability to make high or low responses to some antigens is under genetic control.
2. In the guinea pig the PLL gene is a single, autosomal, dominant gene which controls the recognition of the carrier PLL by T-cells.
3. In mice, genes which control the response to a wide variety of antigens are associated with the H-2 complex. These genes are located in the I region of H-2.
4. The mechanism by which these genes regulate the ability to respond to antigens is unknown and may involve defects in B-cells, T-cells, or both.
5. A suppressor T-cell has been implicated in at least one form of nonresponsiveness.

READINGS

REVIEWS

Benacerraf, B., Green, I., and Paul, W. E. (1967). The immune response of guinea pigs to hapten-poly-L-lysine conjugates as an example of genetic control of the recognition of antigenicity, *Cold Spring Harbor Symposium on Quant. Biol.* **32,** 569. (A review of the PLL gene.)

McDevitt, H. O., and Benacerraf, B. (1969). Genetic control of specific immune responses, *Adv. Immunol.* **11,** 31. (An excellent review of the beginnings of the field.)

Benacerraf, B., and Katz, D. H. (1975). The nature and function of histocompatability-linked immune response genes, in *Immunogenetics and Immunodeficiency,* B. Benacerraf (ed.), London, Medical and Technical Publishing Co. (A creative review which brings together genetic control of responses and cell interactions.)

20

IMMUNOLOGICAL TOLERANCE

OVERVIEW

One of the central questions of immunology is how the body can distinguish self from nonself. As we have seen in all the previous chapters, animals can respond to a wide variety of foreign substances, yet they do not normally respond to their own tissues. This, of course, is essential, since reaction against normal "self" tissue would be calamitous, and it must mean that animals can distinguish self from nonself. Investigation of this intriguing phenomenon has led to the discovery that experimental animals can be manipulated in such a manner that their response to a specific antigen will be suppressed or abolished. This specific suppression is called IMMUNOLOGICAL TOLER-ANCE, a term which derives from the idea that the foreign substance is being tolerated by the immune system as if it were self. As the study of tolerance has progressed, it has become increasingly clear that specific suppression (and in some cases nonspecific suppression) of the immune response may be an integral part of the regulation of the immune response.

This chapter will examine several aspects of immune suppression in the context of both self-recognition and self-regulation. It will be shown that tolerance can be induced in both adult and neonatal animals in both B-cells and T-cells. While the mechanism of tolerance is not clear, deletion of clones and of suppressor cells are likely candidates.

247

INDUCTION OF IMMUNOLOGICAL TOLERANCE

Tolerance in the Newborn

In 1945 R. D. Owen made the remarkable discovery that some nonidentical twin cattle contain a mixture of each other's red blood cells. In these *dizygotic twins* there had been intertwining of the embryonic blood systems before birth which allowed an exchange of the blood of the two embryos. Owen astutely noted that since each of these cattle had red blood cells of its own and its twin's blood type even as an adult, some "embryonal cells ancestral to the erythrocyte" must have been exchanged and survived in the adult.

Burnet and Fenner in 1949 used this observation as a crucial element for a model for self-recognition. They speculated that since embryo P had come in contact with the cells of embryo Q before birth, cells of P were later treated as "self" by Q. This led them to predict that if antigen were introduced into the body early enough in development, the animal would consider it "self" and not react against it. P. B. Medawar and his colleagues successfully carried out exactly this experiment in 1953. They injected embryos of CBA mice with various tissues of A-strain mice. Then, when the CBA animals reached maturity, they grafted skin from strain A and skin of a third strain onto the CBA mice. The third-party skin was rejected as expected, but the A skin was not. In this manner it was treated as self, or "tolerated." This phenomena was called *immunological tolerance*. The experiment is diagrammed in Figure 1. Burnet and Medawar shared the Nobel prize for this work in 1960.

In his Nobel prize lecture Burnet stated that "when Medawar and his colleagues showed that immunological tolerance could be produced experimentally the new immunology was born."

Tolerance in the Adult

With the discovery that specific nonresponsiveness to tissue antigens could be induced by intrauterine or neonatal injection, many investigators attempted to induce tolerance to protein and other antigens in a similar manner in both newborns and adults. One of the most striking examples of induction of tolerance to a protein in *adults* was obtained with bovine gamma globulin (BGG) as antigen. If BGG is ultracentrifuged to remove molecular aggregates, the remaining aggregate-free antigen, when injected into adult mice, is able to induce a state of specific unresponsiveness or tolerance. A typical experiment of this kind is shown in Figure 2. The tolerance is specific (as it was in tolerance to tissues) since the animals make normal responses to an antigen with which they were not pretreated. The tolerance-inducing antigen is called the TOLEROGEN, and the challeng-

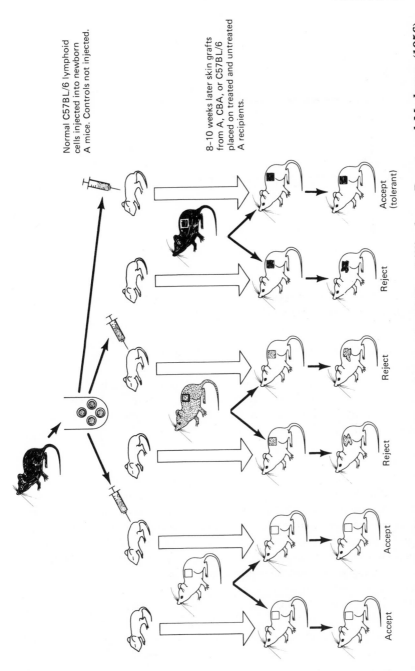

Normal C57BL/6 lymphoid cells injected into newborn A mice. Controls not injected.

8–10 weeks later skin grafts from A, CBA, or C57BL/6 placed on treated and untreated A recipients.

Accept (tolerant)

Reject

Reject

Reject

Accept

Accept

The induction of tolerance to tissues in newborn mice. [After Billingham, Brent, and Medawar (1956). *Phil. Trans. Royal Soc. B* **239, 357.**]

1

2

Removal of molecular aggregates of BGG converts it into a tolerogen.
[**After Dresser (1962).** *Immunology,* **5, 161.**]

ing antigen (to which controls respond normally) is called the IM-
MUNOGEN.

In the above examples we saw that antigen introduced into very
young animals or aggregate-free antigen injected into the adult
induced tolerance. There are a variety of other means of inducing
tolerance in adults.

Radiomimetic Drugs

Treatment with drugs which interfere with the immune response
at the same time that antigen is given can result in a state of
tolerance to the antigen. An example of this is seen in Figure 3 where
the drug is the alkylating agent cyclophosphamide. This drug inter-
feres with the replication of DNA in a manner which mimics radiation (for this reason it is called a *radiomimetic* drug). In the experiment the drug was used to induce tolerance to SRBC. Cyclophosphamide was injected into mice at various times before the injection
of SRBC or at times after the animals were injected with SRBC. All
the mice received SRBC on days 7, 14, 21, and 28 and were assayed
for anti-SRBC antibodies on day 25. As is readily seen from the
figure, treatment with the drug 7 or 14 days before SRBC injection
had no effect on subsequent SRBC responses. However, treatment for
a narrow time span of 3 days before or 3 days after SRBC treatment

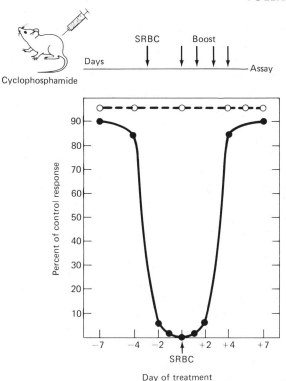

Mice were treated with cyclophosphamide either before or after receiving SRBC as tolerogen. SRBC were injected several times, and anti-SRBC assayed on day 35. Anti-SRBC response was diminished, but response to non-cross-reacting antigen was normal. [From Aisenberg (1967). *J. Exp. Med.* 125, 833.]

3

resulted in loss of ability to produce anti-SRBC while the ability to respond to an unrelated antigen was unimpaired. This shows that a state of specific tolerance was established to SRBC when the radiomimetic drug was used at the time that antigen was introduced. Similar results have been obtained with BSA in the rabbit using not only radiomimetic drugs but nonlethal doses of X-irradiation.

Antigen Form

The form in which the antigen is injected can also be important in inducing immunity or tolerance. If the antigen is in a form to which the animal cannot respond by producing antibody or a cell-mediated response, a state of tolerance is often established. We have already seen that the aggregate-free form of the antigen induces tolerance. Another example of this is seen when mice are injected with the hapten DNP on a carrier which is nonimmunogenic such as poly-D-GL. This is a random polymer of D-glutamic acid and D-lysine. The L-polymer of poly-GL is immunogenic, but the D-polymer is not. When mice pretreated with the DNP-D-GL polymer are challenged with DNP on the immunogenic carrier KLH, they fail to produce antibody to DNP but make normal amounts of antibody to an unrelated antigen. Thus the DNP-D-GL acts as a tolerogen.

Antigen Concentration

Another means of inducing tolerance is to treat animals with *extremes of antigen concentration*. In a phenomenon known as *immune paralysis* discovered by Felton in 1934, mice are treated with either 100 or $10\mu g$ pneumococcal polysaccharide (abbreviated S III). The mice which receive the $10\mu g$ S III are protected when challenged with virulent pneumococcus organisms, but all those pretreated with $100\mu g$ die of the disease. In this case a low dose immunized the mice, but a high dose did not. It was thought that the high dose of antigen "paralysed" the immune system. We now think of this as a form of tolerance in which there is failure of lymphocytes to respond to antigen.

A rather surprising observation was made when *extremely low doses* of protein antigen were used to induce tolerance. In the heroic experiment of Mitchison shown in Figure 4 groups of mice were injected with varying doses of soluble BSA three times a week for up to 16 weeks. In this way the effect of dose and time could be determined. The animals were then challenged with the immunogenic form of BSA, and anti-BSA antibody titers were determined. When the data was plotted, it was found that high doses of tolerogen induced tolerance (as expected) but that very low doses also induced tolerance. This phenomenon is called LOW ZONE TOLERANCE and has now been observed with several antigens. Treatment with middle doses of BSA primed the mice.

Antibody-Induced Tolerance

Tolerance can also be induced by administrating *antibody*. Antibody-mediated tolerance may have a regulatory role in the immune response. This form of tolerance has been studied both *in vivo* and *in vitro*. An example of an *in vivo* experiment is outlined in Figure 5. In this study varying amounts of anti-polymerized flagellin (anti-POL) antibody were added to cultures of normal spleen cells. The cultures were then immunized to either POL or SRBC. The

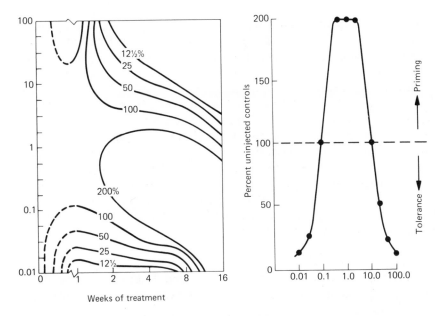

Weeks of treatment

High- and low-zone tolerances. "Contour" map on left; 2-week treatment data on right. See text for details. [From Mitchison (1964). *Proc. Royal Soc. B.* 161, 275.]

SRBC antigen serves as a specificity control in these experiments since the treatment of the cultures with anti-POL should have no effect on an SRBC response if tolerance is specific. It can be seen that increasing the concentration of anti-POL in the cultures inhibits a POL response but has no effect on an SRBC response. This specific suppression by definition is tolerance. How the antibody acts in preventing a specific response in antibody-mediated tolerance has not yet been resolved. Most cellular immunologists feel that the mode of action is "afferent," i.e., by binding antigen and thus preventing it from reacting with receptors on lymphocytes. A body of data exists, however, which argues for a "central" mechanism, i.e., that the antibody reacts with the antigen-reactive cell preventing it (in some unknown way) from responding to antigen.

INDUCTION OF TOLERANCE IN B- AND T-CELLS

In the section above we saw that the tolerant state can be induced in a variety of ways; a very important question is whether both T-cells and B-cells can be made tolerant. In the very straightforward experiment of Chiller and his co-workers seen in Figure 6, it was shown that both helper T-cells and B-cells can be rendered tolerant. In this experiment mice were injected with human gamma globulin (HGG) which had been made aggregate-free. At varying days after this treatment with antigen the mice were sacrificed, and their thymus and bone marrow cells harvested. Thymus cells from the treated mice were injected into irradiated recipients along with bone marrow from normal mice. Bone marrow from treated mice was injected along with normal thymus cells. Thymus and bone marrow from normal mice served as controls. The groups which received thymus *or* bone marrow from treated mice were tolerant. This shows that there are no functional helper cells for HGG in the thymus of tolerant mice and that there are no functional effector B-cells for anti-HGG production in the bone marrow of tolerant mice.

Kinetics of Tolerance
    Having established that both B-cells and T-cells can be rendered tolerant, the same investigators then showed that T-cells are more

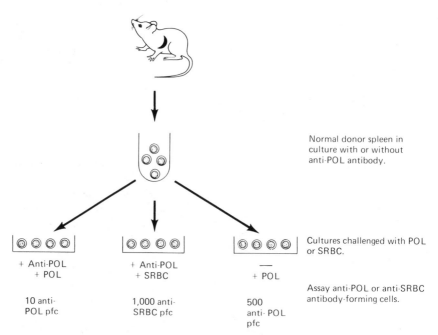

Induction of tolerance *in vitro* to POL by the addition of anti-POL antibody to the cultures. [After Feldmann and Diener (1970). *J. Exp. Med.* 131, 247.]

Induction of tolerance in bone marrow and thymus cells. [**After Chiller** *et al.* **(1971).** *Science,* **171, 831.**]

quickly made tolerant than B-cells. This was shown by repopulating irradiated recipients with combinations of normal or tolerant bone marrow or thymus cells as in Figure 6. The experiment was varied by using as donors mice which had been injected with tolerogen at varying days before sacrifice. In this way thymus cells from a donor injected 1 day, 2 days, etc., earlier were combined with normal bone marrow so that the time taken for the population of cells in the thymus to be rendered tolerant could be determined. Similar experiments with bone marrow were also carried out. It was found that thymus cells became tolerant very rapidly (by 2 days) but that bone marrow cells became tolerant more slowly (by 10 days).

MECHANISMS OF TOLERANCE

Clonal Deletion

Not long ago it was thought that research would establish one mechanism of tolerance. This hopeful state was the result of thinking that we were about to bring all the problems of B-cells, T-cells and macrophages into one grand unifying concept of how the immune response works. Today we know that there are probably multiple mechanisms of tolerance induction because there probably are multiple mechanisms by which B-cells, T-cells, and macrophages interact. The original notion of the mechanism of tolerance was *clonal deletion*. It was thought that antigen reacted with a lymphocyte surface receptor, and because of the form of the antigen or the state of the lymphocyte, either induction of an immune response or induction of tolerance occurred. As the role of T-cells as helper cells and B-cells as antibody producers became evident, it also became clear that there might be different mechanisms of tolerance induction in each population. We do not know if specific antigen-reactive clones of cells are actually deleted in tolerance or if they are present but not able to respond to immunogenic antigen.

One of the earliest ideas about tolerance was Burnet's notion that lymphoid cells early in differentiation should be rendered tolerant more easily than in adults and be eliminated. There is some experimental basis for such an idea. In experiments where F_1 hosts are repopulated with parental spleen cells, if the donors of the spleen cells were neonatally thymectomized, their spleen cells are able to recolonize an irradiated F_1 with no GVH reaction. The lack of mature donor T-cells after neonatal thymectomy allows the recipients to survive with no acute GVH reactions because there are no host T-cells which could have recirculated into the bone marrow. No chronic or long-term GVH reaction develops because the cells that migrate to the thymus to become thymocytes and T-cells become tolerant. If this is the reason, the best present interpretation of these experiments seems to be that T-cells are more easily rendered tolerant early in their differentiation than late in differentiation. In the examples cited, it is thought that the young T-cells which begin to differentiate in the F_1 react with host antigen in the environment and are rendered tolerant. We do not know if this is due to clonal deletion, but it seems that these experiments may be dealing with a mechanism of self-tolerance. A similar observation using *in vitro* cloning procedures has been made. In these experiments spleen cells from neonatal mice are rendered tolerant to a hapten much more readily than cells from adults.

Antigen-Binding Cells in Tolerant Animals

One way of approaching the question of deletion of clones has been to look for *antigen-binding cells* after tolerance induction. If clones of antigen-reactive cells are eliminated, then the number of cells able to bind antigen specifically would be expected to decrease. It will be remembered from Chapter 10 that both B-cells and T-cells can be shown to react specifically with antigen. If clonal deletion is really a mechanism of tolerance, then one might expect that there would be no cells able to bind the antigen to which the animal is tolerant. The results of these kinds of experiments have been rather variable, but most investigators have found that antigen-binding cells are not eliminated in tolerance, raising questions about clonal deletion as a mechanism of tolerance. But even when the number of antigen-binding cells is not diminished, we do not know that the cells which bind the antigen can actually respond to it. Recently, for example, it has been shown with the tolerogen DNP-D-GL that the tolerogen seems to immobilize the membrane. It could be that one mechanism of tolerance is the "freezing" of the membrane by tolerogenic antigen so that the clone would be *functionally deleted* but still physically present.

Suppressor Cells in Tolerance

In Chapter 18 we dealt extensively with the regulatory role of the T-cell through its function as a suppressor cell. Since the almost universal realization of the existence of the suppressor T-cell, there have been a good many experiments trying to identify suppressor T-cells in tolerance to various antigens. Suppressor cells playing a role in tolerance to contact sensitivity to picryl chloride and in antibody formation to BGG and SRBC have been reported. But inability to find suppressor cells in tolerance in antibody formation has also been claimed. It is clear that we are early into the era of the suppressor cell, and the role, if any, of this cell in the induction or maintenance of tolerance remains to be determined.

NONSPECIFIC SUPPRESSION: ANTIGENIC COMPETITION

So far all the suppression which we have dealt with in this chapter has been antigen-specific. There is another, very poorly understood, form of suppression which is not antigen-specific and is called AN-TIGENIC COMPETITION. If an antigen (X) is given to an animal and another antigen (Y) is given soon after, the response to Y is often significantly depressed. An example of this is seen in Figure 7 where

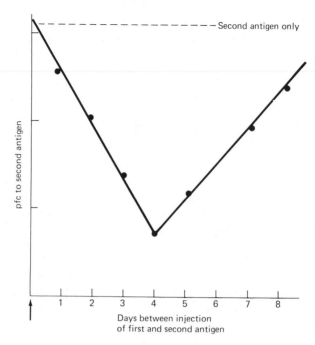

7

Antigenic competition. Response to second antigen is reduced if second antigen is given after first antigen. (↑) = injection of first antigen. [After Radovitch and Talmadge (1967). *Science*, 158, 512.]

mice were injected with SRBC at day 0, and then groups were injected with a second, non-cross-reacting antigen, HRBC, at varying days after the first injection. Antibody-forming cells to HRBC (the second antigen) were then determined. It can be seen in the figure that when there is a 4-day interval between the injection of antigen X (SRBC) and antigen Y (HRBC), the response to Y is depressed. Clearly this form of immune suppression is not antigen specific since it is the second antigen which is depressed, and virtually any antigen given as the second antigen would be depressed. In other words, the specific response to one antigen causes a nonspecific depression of the response to the second.

The phenomenon of antigenic competition is of practical importance in vaccines. If mixtures of immunogens are inoculated, will the response to one antigen be impaired because of the presence of the others? Unfortunately there is very little yet in the way of explanation of the phenomenon of antigenic competition. Investigators have

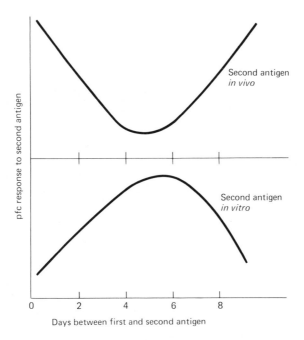

Paradoxical response to second antigen given *in vivo* (upper curve) or *in vitro* (lower curve) after injection of first antigen. First antigen was *in vivo* in both cases. [After Waterson (1970). *Science,* 170, 1108.]

postulated a wide variety of mechanisms including humoral suppressive factors, competition for nutrients, competition for a limiting cell type, production of suppressor cells, and other things too horrible to contemplate.

The difficulties of studying antigenic competition are exemplified in the experiment in Figure 8. Groups of mice were immunized with SRBC as the first antigen. The second antigen, pig RBC (PRBC), was either injected *in vivo* or the spleen cells put in culture and the antigen added *in vitro*. The totally *in vivo* groups gave pfc responses similar to those in Figure 7, i.e., a depression of the response to the second antigen. But the groups which were challenged with the second antigen *in vitro* showed a significant *increase* in pfc to PRBC instead of a decrease. The title of the paper in which this experiment was presented was "Antigen Competition: A Paradox." This statement eloquently summarizes the status of our understanding of antigenic competition.

SUMMARY

1. Immunological tolerance is the inability of an animal to generate an immune response against a specific antigen while making normal responses to other antigens.
2. Tolerance can be induced by injecting antigen into the newborn animal or in the adult by using antigen in nonimmunogenic form, by the addition of antibody, by extremes of antigen concentration, or in conjunction with certain drugs or X-ray.
3. Both B-cells and T-cells are tolerant in a tolerant animal, but they become tolerant at different rates.
4. The mechanism of tolerance is not known. Deletion of specific clones and the induction of suppressor cells are possible mechanisms. The number of cells able to bind the specific antigen does not decrease greatly in a tolerant animal, but it is not known if these cells are functional.
5. Antigenic competition is the nonspecific suppression of the response to a second antigen given shortly after injection of the first antigen. The mechanism is not known.

READINGS

BOOKS AND REVIEWS

Landy, M., and Braun, W. (1969). *Immunological Tolerance. A Reassessment of Mechanisms of the Immune Response,* New York, Academic.

Katz, D. H., and Benacerraf, B. (1974). *Immunological Tolerance. Mechanisms and Potential Therapeutic Applications,* New York, Academic.

Golub, E. S. (1975). Cellular immunology today, *Science,* **187,** 1069. (Book review which compares and contrasts the two symposium volumes above.)

Weigle, W. O. (1967). *Natural and Acquired Immunologic Unresponsiveness,* Cleveland, World Publishing. (A pre-B- and T-cell monograph.)

Billingham, R. E., Brent, L., and Medawar, P. B. (1956). Quantitative studies on tissue transplantation immunity. III. Activity acquired tolerance, *Phil. Trans. B.* **239,** 257.

Dresser, D. W. (1962). Specific inhibition of antibody production. II. Paralysis induced in adult mice by small quantities of protein antigen, *Immunology,* **5,** 378. (Aggregate-free antigen acts as tolerogen.)

Mitchison, N. A. (1965). Induction of immunological paralysis in two zones of dosage, *Proc. Roy. Soc. Ser. B.* **161,** 275. (High- and low-zone tolerance.)

Chiller, J. M., Habicht, G. S., and Weigle, W. O. (1971). Kinetic differences in unresponsiveness of thymus and bone marrow cells, *Science,* **171,** 813.

APPENDICES

APPENDIX I. THE NATURE OF IMMUNE REACTIONS

When an antigen is injected, or in some cases ingested, or comes into contact with the skin, a very complex series of cellular events follows. The result of these events is the production of antibodies or the generation of cell-mediated responses. How these two reactions are initiated by antigen is the subject matter of the text. In this Appendix we will describe some very rudimentary aspects of the measurement of immune reactions. To determine if an animal has made an immune response, we can measure the reaction to the antigen either *in vivo* or *in vitro*. Since the immune response is specific, the response will be directed only toward the antigen used to immunize the animal. In this context *specificity* means preferential reaction of the antibody or cells of an immunized animal with the antigen used to elicit the response. The magnitude of an immune response is always a measure of the amount of reaction with the specific antigen.

ANTIBODY REACTIONS

Antigen-Antibody Reaction

The interaction of antigen and antibody can be looked upon as a chemical reaction in which two reactants come together and form a product. Thus:

$$Ag + Ab \rightleftharpoons AgAb$$

In this equation Ag is the antigen and Ab is the antibody. The product, AgAb, is called the ANTIGEN-ANTIBODY COMPLEX. The antigen-antibody reaction results in the formation of the Ag-Ab complex. Since the Ag-Ab complex is the product of the reaction of antigen and antibody, the *quantity* formed or the *rate* at which it is formed is used as a means of determining the concentration of antibodies to a certain antigen in a sample.

Methods to Quantitate Antibodies

The *precipitation reaction* is used to determine the quantity of antibody present when the antigen used is a *soluble* one. Typical soluble antigens are proteins such as *albumins* (e.g., bovine serum albumin, BSA; ovalbumin, OA), *globulins* (e.g., human gamma globulin, HGG; bovine gamma globulin, BGG), or proteins such as keyhole limpet hemocyanin (KLH). These antigens are termed *soluble* because they remain in solution. However, when reacted with antibody, complexes of antigen and antibody are formed which become larger and larger and precipitate out of solution. This happens because most antigens are *multivalent;* that is, they have many antigenic determinants, and so several antibody molecules can bind to them. Since most antibody molecules are at least *bivalent,* i.e., have two binding sites per molecule, a very large complex may form which, as it grows, begins to precipitate out of solution. The amount of precipitate which forms is used as a measure of the amount of antibody present.

When the antigen is *particulate,* i.e., too large to stay in solution, a variant of the precipitation reaction, called the *agglutination reaction,* is used to quantitate the amount of antibody in a sample. Examples of commonly used particulate antigens are red blood cells (RBC) and bacteria. Since these particles settle out of solution by themselves, the mere act of settling to the bottom of the tube cannot be used, as in the precipitation reaction, to determine the presence of an Ag-Ab complex. However, particulate antigens show a different *pattern* of settling out of solution when they have reacted with antibody. The Ag-Ab reaction causes clumps or agglutinates to form, and these look different than normally settled particulate antigen.

Qualitative Vs. Quantitative Measurements

The amount of antibody can be determined as either an absolute or a relative value. For a relative value the exact quantity (in terms of grams of protein or number of molecules) in a sample is not determined; instead, only the fact that there is x times more in one sample than in another is determined. This is done by determining how far the sample of antibody can be diluted and still give a measurable antigen-antibody complex. As an example, two samples of anti-BSA are diluted 1/2, 1/4, 1/8, etc., to 1/256. This means that each dilution has half the quantity of material as the preceding one. Such dilutions are called SERIAL dilutions (in this case serial twofold dilutions). A constant amount of BSA is added to each dilution, and the mixture of antigen and antibody is incubated for several hours before being examined for the presence of precipitate. If one sample still forms precipitate at 1/128 and the other forms precipitate only to a dilution of 1/8, we know that the first sample had more antibody than the second because we could get a measurable reaction after lowering the concentration of antibody in each sample by dilution. Since a 1/128 dilution required four more twofold dilutions, we can say that there is approximately eight times more antibody in one than the other (4 × 2, the dilution factor). We still do not know how much antibody is in either sample, but we do know that one sample has more than the other.

Immunology began to enter the modern quantitative age in 1935 when Michael Heidelberger invented the *quantitative precipitation reaction*. The historical importance of this contribution cannot be emphasized enough because at that point immunology became a quantitative science. The quantitative precipitation reaction consists of measuring the amount of nitrogen in the precipitate and allows the antigen-antibody reaction to be expressed as milligrams per milliliter of antibody in a sample rather than as the relative titer.

Precipitation Reactions in Gels

The qualitative and quantitative precipitation reactions are carried out in liquid, and the presence or quantity of the precipitate is determined. If more than one antigen-antibody complex were to be formed, this fact could not be distinguished from a single Ag-Ab complex. To visualize more than one reaction and begin to characterize the nature of cross reactions, a method was developed by Ouchterlony in which the precipitation reaction is carried out in a solid supporting medium. In this reaction wells are cut in agar, and each well is filled with either antigen or antibody. The molecules diffuse toward each other at rates which are unique to each antigen, and they reach the optimal proportion of antigen and antibody to form a complex and precipitate at different places in the gel. Different antigen-antibody systems diffuse at different rates and precipitate at different places in the gel. Patterns of reaction can show partial sharing of antigenic determinants on an antigen molecule.

A useful modification of this method is *immunoelectrophoresis* which combines electrophoresis and precipitation in gels. Since most antigen molecules carry a net charge, they can migrate in an electric field (i.e., an electrophoretic separation is possible). If the electric field is applied across a gel, the molecules will move in the gel and be immobilized at the point to which they have migrated. If antibody is now added to a trough cut in the gel, an antigen-antibody complex will form and precipitate at the point where the antigen has migrated. This is especially useful when complex mixtures of antigens are used.

COMPLEMENT

COMPLEMENT (C) is a series of proteins found in normal serum which have the ability to react sequentially with an antigen-antibody complex. This sequential reaction is called the COMPLEMENT CASCADE. It is initiated when one component of complement reacts with the Fc portion of an antibody molecule when that antibody molecule has bound an antigen in its antigen-combining site. If the antibody has not reacted with antigen, C will not be bound. One of the components of C is an enzyme which causes holes to be made in membranes. If the antigen is a cell (an erythrocyte or bacterial cell, for example), the combination of Ag-Ab and C will disrupt the membrane and cause the cell to burst or *lyse*.

Since C binds (or fixes) only to antigen-antibody complexes, it can be used to quantitate the amount of complex formed. This can be done in either of two ways. If the antigen is a cell, the amount of lysis which the antibody causes can be measured and will reflect the amount of antibody bound to the cells. The other method is to determine the amount of C bound to the Ag-Ab complex indirectly by allowing a known amount of C to react with the Ag-Ab complex and then to measure the amount of the added C which has not been bound to the complex. This method is called the QUANTITATIVE COMPLEMENT FIXATION REACTION (see below).

Because complement lyses cells which are coated with antibody, it is a very important part of the defense system against bacterial infection. If invading bacteria induce an antibody response and become coated with antibody, the complement in the serum and body fluids can cause them to lyse. The C components compose almost 10 percent of normal serum globulins in mammals. These proteins react with virtually all Ag-Ab complex, and so no antigen specificity is involved.

Hemolysis and C-Fixation Reactions

C fixes to Ag-Ab complexes forming an Ag-Ab-C complex, and if the Ag is a cell, the cell will be lysed. If the cell is an erythrocyte, hemoglobin is released after lysis. This is called HEMOLYSIS. By measuring the amount of hemoglobin liberated, one has a measure of the amount of hemolysis and thus of the amount of Ag-Ab complex.

Complement *fixation* takes advantage of the fact that C fixes to Ag-Ab complexes. The amount of C in a sample of normal serum is determined by first diluting the C and adding preformed Ag-Ab complexes of RBC-anti-RBC to the diluted samples. (In this way the C concentration is titrated.) An aliquot of this C with known titer is then added to a mixture of the antigen and antibody which is being tested. If an Ag-Ab complex forms, some of the added C will react with the complex. The point of the quantitative complement-fixation reaction is to measure the amount of C remaining in the sample.

To measure the residual unreacted C, RBC-anti-RBC complex is added to the remaining C and the amount of hemolysis is measured. If the unknown sample of antigen and antibody formed no Ag-Ab complexes, then all the added C remains and the test RBC-anti-system is lysed. If there was antibody in the unknown sample, it would react with Ag to form Ag-Ab complexes, and some of the added C would bind to the complex and not be available to react with the RBC-anti-RBC complex when it is added later.

Hemolytic Plaque Assay

The assay which is referred to more than any other in this text is the *hemolytic plaque assay*. This assay, developed by Niels Jerne in 1963, is to the study of the cellular basis of the immune reaction what the quantitative precipitation reaction is to immunochemistry. The hemolytic plaque assay measures the number of antibody-forming cells in a population. These cells are usually expressed as *plaque-forming cells* (pfc). The principle of the plaque assay is that if the cells producing antibody against an erythrocyte antigen are suspended in an agar layer containing the erythrocyte antigens, the antibody secreted by a single cell will diffuse through the agar and react with the erythrocytes, forming localized antigen-antibody complexes. When complement is added to the erythrocyte-lymphocyte layer, only those erythrocytes which have reacted with antibody will fix complement and be lysed. This results in localized areas of hemolysis. These local areas are called *plaques* because they resemble the plaques in a bacteriophage assay. (Here is another case of the influence of the phage group on Jerne's thinking. The philosophical contribution of Max Delbrück and his colleagues of the phage group to modern biology are so widespread that decades will probably pass before its real magnitude can be accurately judged.)

Pfc are quantitated as plaques per spleen, plaques per culture, or plaques per 10^6 tested cells. The method gives a quantitative measure of the cells producing antibody against an antigen. By conjugating proteins or small molecules called *haptens* to the erythrocytes, the pfc against a fairly wide variety of antigens can be determined.

CELL-MEDIATED RESPONSES

One of the main themes of this text is that the immune response is made up of both an antibody and a cell-mediated response. Cell-mediated reactions are those in which antibody does not play a role. They are usually tissue-destroying reactions in which sensitized cells carry out the damage without the use of antibody. The body of the text goes into great detail about the cellular basis of these two types of reactions. In fact, the three basic cell-mediated responses which are used in the experiments in the text are described in Chapter 4. Here we will briefly describe some of the more common cell-mediated reactions.

Delayed-Type Hypersensitivity

The most common *in vivo* cell-mediated reaction is *delayed-type hypersensitivity* (DTH). In DTH reactions the animal is sensitized with an initial injection of the antigen. After a suitable interval the antigen is injected into the skin. A local reaction occurs at the site of the injection, and the magnitude of this local reaction is measured after 48 hr. The swelling at the site can be measured with a caliper. The site can be the skin on the flank of the animal or, in the mouse, the foot pad or the ear. An alternative method is to deposit antigen into the foot pad or ear of a sensitized mouse and then inject either radiolabeled BSA or ^{125}IUdR. The concentrations of isotope at the site are then measured and correlate very well with measurements of swelling.

In Vitro Methods

The two most commonly used *in vitro* cell-mediated responses are the *mixed lymphocyte reaction* (MLR) and *cell-mediated lympholysis* (CML). Both of these reactions measure the responses of one kind of lymphocyte (the T-cell) to antigens present on the surface of cells.

In the MLR the ability of a cell surface antigen to cause a cell to *proliferate* is measured. This is done by mixing the test lymphocytes with lymphocytes of another individual or strain of mouse. After 2 days tritiated thymidine is added to the culture, and the amount of label incorporated into DNA is determined. There is a high correlation between the amount of cell replication and incorporation of nucleotide into DNA.

In the CML reaction the response of T-cells to antigen on another cell is measured by the ability of the sensitized T-cell to lyse a radiolabeled target cell. The target cell has the same surface antigens that the stimulating cell had, and so one is measuring the number of *cytotoxic* or *killer cells* which have been generated in response to the antigenic stimulus. It is seen in Chapters 4 and 8 that these are two separate reactions rather than two manifestations of the same basic phenomenon.

APPENDIX II. SURFACE PROPERTIES OF SUBPOPULATIONS OF T-CELLS

In the text evidence was presented for the existence of several subpopulations of T-cells. A nomenclature which appears to be gaining wide acceptance is to identify the T-cell subpopulation by its function. Hence, helper T-cells are termed T_H, suppressor T-cells T_S, etc. Table 1 compares Ly and Ia antigens on the various T-cell subpopulations.

TABLE 1. SURFACE ANTIGENS ON FUNCTIONAL T-CELL SUBCLASSES.*

	T-Cell Subclass			
	Helper (T_H)	*Cytotoxic* (T_C)	*Delayed* *hypersensitivity* (T_{DT})	*Suppressor* (T_S)
Theta	+	+	+	+
Ly	1	2,3	1	2,3
Ia	(IA–B)	–	–	(I–J)
Antigen reactivity	Carrier, LD	SD	SD	?

*The functions of the Ly 1, 2, 3 cells, called T_E (embryonic), are not known.

269

GLOSSARY

Adherent cell A nonlymphoid cell which adheres to plastic or glass. Syn. macrophage.

Allelic exclusion The synthesis of Ig of only one parental allotype by an F_1 lymphocyte.

Allogeneic Genetically different members of the same species.

Allogeneic effect The overcoming of the carrier effect by an allogeneic reaction.

Allotype Antigens on Ig molecules coded at one genetic locus and inherited as alleles.

B-cell Ig^+, θ^- lymphocyte of bursal origin which is the effector cell in antibody formation.

β-2 microglobulin Small peptide associated with H-2 and HLA.

Bence-Jones protein Light chain secreted in urine of patients with multiple myeloma.

Bursa of Fabricius The inducing microenvironment for B-cells in birds.

Capping see Patching.

Carrier determinants The determinants on an antigen which react with T helper cells.

Carrier effect The need for an identical carrier molecule on which hapten is coupled for both primary and secondary antihapten responses.

CML Cell-Mediated Lympholysis. Killing of labeled target cells by sensitized T-cells.

Chimera Cells of different genetic origins existing in one individual.

Complement Series of interacting serum proteins which combine with antigen-antibody complexes and cause lysis of cells.

ConA Concanavalin A. T-cell mitogen.

Congenic mice Mice which are identical in all but a few defined genes.

Constant region Area of Ig molecules with amino acid sequences similar to other Ig molecules.

C receptor Complement receptor on lymphocytes.

DTH Delayed-type hypersensitivity. Cell-mediated reaction measured as skin reaction.

E-rosettes Cluster of sheep RBC around a human T lymphocyte.

Germ line theory Theory of generation of diversity which postulates that the information for antibody specificity is passed through germ cells (sperm and egg).

GVH Graft-versus-host reaction. Cell-mediated reaction in which T-cells in grafted tissue react with antigens of the host.

Haplotype Set of genetic determinants coded by closely linked genes on a single chromosome.

H chain   Heavy chain of immunoglobulins.

Helper cell   Subpopulation of T-cells which cooperate with precursors of effector cells.

Hemolysis   The disintegration (lysis) of an erythrocyte.

Hemopoiesis   The process of blood cell formation.

Humoral   Pertaining to antibody responses.

Ia antigens   I-associated antigens. Serologically defined antigens coded in the I region of H-2.

Idiotype   Antigenic marker of the antigen-combining site on an immunoglobulin molecule.

Ig   Immunoglobulin.

IgT   Ig associated with thymus-derived lymphocytes.

Indirect plaque assay   Method for detecting IgG antibody producing cells.

Ir genes   Genes in the I region of H-2 which control antibody responses.

Isoantibodies   Antibodies produced by one member of a species against antigen of another member of the same species.

Isoantigens   Antigens of one member of a species which can elicit antibody in another member of the same species.

Isogeneic   Of the same genetic constitution (see allogeneic and xenogeneic).

J protein   Peptide which binds monomeric units in polymeric IgA and IgM.

L chain   Light chain of Ig.

LD antigens   Lymphocyte defined antigens coded in the I region of H-2 and expressed preferentially on lymphocytes.

LPS   Bacterial lipopolysaccharide. B-cell mitogen.

Ly antigens   Allelic antigens expressed by subpopulation of T-cells.

Lymphokines   Biologically active molecules produced by lymphocytes.

Macrophage   Nonlymphoid accessory cell important in immune function.

MHC   Major histocompatability complex. H-2 in mouse and HLA in man.

MIF   Migration inhibition factor. Product of the T-cell which inhibits the migration of macrophages.

Mitogen   Substance which induces cells to enter mitosis.

MLR   Mixed lymphocyte reaction. Induction of proliferation by T-cells after recognition of antigen on another lymphocyte.

Myeloma   Tumor of Ig secreting cell.

Myeloma proteins   Ig products of myelomas.

NK cell   Natural killer cell. Cell able to kill tumors without prior sensitization.

Nude mouse   Congenitally athymic mouse.

Null cell   Lymphocyte without B-cell or T-cell surface markers.

Patching   (and capping) the movement of molecules in the plane of the lymphocyte membrane.

PHA   Phytohemagglutinin. T-cell mitogen.

Primary lymphoid organs   Thymus and bursa or bone marrow; site of lymphopoiesis.

Private specificities   Serologically defined H-2 antigens unique to a haplotype.

Public specificities   Serologically defined H-2 antigens shared by strains of several haplotypes.

SD antigens   Serologically defined antigens of the K and D regions of H-2.

Secondary lymphoid organs   Peripheral concentrations of lymphocytes; spleen and lymph nodes.

Splenomegaly   The increase in size of the spleen as a result of a GVH reaction.

T-cell   Thymus-derived lymphocyte in the peripheral lymphoid organs.

Theta antigen θ or Thy 1. Alloantigen unique to thymus-derived lymphocytes.

Thymocyte   Lymphocyte of the thymus.

TL antigen   Thymus leukemia antigen. A differentiation alloantigen on thymocytes.

Tolerance   Inability to respond to a specific antigen.

Xenogeneic   Members of different species.

INDEX

273